Against-Medical-Advice Discharges from the Hospital

David Alfandre
Editor

Against-Medical-Advice Discharges from the Hospital

Optimizing Prevention and Management to
Promote High Quality, Patient-Centered Care

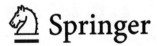 Springer

Editor
David Alfandre
VHA National Center for Ethics in Health Care
Department of Veterans Affairs
NYU School of Medicine
New York, NY, USA

ISBN 978-3-319-75129-0   ISBN 978-3-319-75130-6   (eBook)
https://doi.org/10.1007/978-3-319-75130-6

Library of Congress Control Number: 2018939065

Printed on acid-free paper

This Springer imprint is published by the registered company Springer International Publishing AG part of Springer Nature.
The registered company address is: Gewerbestrasse 11, 6330 Cham, Switzerland

"You may not be able to stop nothing from happening. But you got to let him know you's there."

– James Baldwin, "Sonny's Blues"

Preface

A book devoted exclusively to against medical advice (AMA) discharges has been a long time coming. AMA discharges have been a regular clinical practice by health-care professionals since at least the middle of the twentieth century. Currently within the academic literature, there are approximately 811 articles indexed in PubMed devoted to the topic of which half were published since 2008. Although this represents increasing interest in the academic literature, a book dedicated to the topic of AMA discharges has not been published before.

This book is intended for a wide academic and clinical audience interested in AMA discharges as a health-care quality problem. Physicians and other health-care professionals, from nurses, to trainees, to social workers and allied health professionals report a disproportionate amount of time and attention in caring for patients who choose to leave the hospital AMA. They experience frustration, anxiety, and sometimes helplessness when confronted with patients that decline recommended care. This book has been written for them. Hospital administrators, clinical department chairs, and hospital quality managers report the challenges of promoting patient-centered care for all of their patients, while simultaneously attempting to improve the quality of care for vulnerable patients discharged AMA, a vulnerable population with higher morbidity and increased but ineffective use of health-care services. This book has been also written for them. Teaching faculty at medical, nursing, and allied health schools and clinician leaders who supervise the teaching of students and trainees are uncertain how best to model high quality care at the bedside for a difficult-to-help population that intermittently declines recommended care. This book is also for them. Finally, health services researchers have directed their efforts at better understanding and addressing AMA discharges for decades. During that time, the overall AMA rate has increased, and there are almost no evidence-based interventions designed to reduce the morbidity and health services associated with AMA discharges. This book is for them as well.

Although there are multiple professional audiences that will find this book helpful, my hope is that this publication will ultimately benefit patients. For patients who struggle to access and engage with hospital care and are discharged AMA, who have higher rates of morbidity and mortality, and who report feeling stigmatized and sometimes abandoned when receiving health care, the system owes them better care. At the same time, health-care professionals, administrators, educators, and researchers are collectively working to better serve this vulnerable population. We hope then, that by improving health-care professional's understanding, knowledge, attitudes, and abilities, this book ultimately helps patients.

A task this large can only be accomplished with the support of many. I am grateful for the diligence and thoughtfulness of the entire book's contributing authors. Without their continuing dedication and support, this book would not have been possible. Thank you to all of the editorial staff at Springer publishing who made this process easier than it should have been. I am indebted to my many colleagues and collaborators who have been formative in helping to develop the ideas contained in this book: Drs. Michael Yin, Peter Gordon, Marilena Lekas, Lauris Kaldjian, Leonard Feldman, John Henning Schumann, Scott Sherman, David Goldfarb, Eberechukwu Onukwugha, and my colleagues at the VA National Center for Ethics in Health Care. These colleagues are a source of continuing inspiration. Finally, I am deeply grateful to my most important collaborator, my spouse, Joanna Steinglass, MD, who, among other things, is also the finest clinician I know.

New York, NY, USA   David Alfandre

Contents

Contributors

David Alfandre, MD, MSPH VHA National Center for Ethics in Health Care, Department of Veterans Affairs, NYU School of Medicine, New York, NY, USA

Nicole Allen, MD Department of Psychiatry, Lenox Hill Hospital, New York, NY, USA

Armand H. Matheny Antommaria, MD, PhD Department of Pediatrics, Cincinnati Children's Hospital Medical Center, Cincinnati, OH, USA

Jeffrey T. Berger, MD Division of Palliative Medicine and Bioethics, Department of Medicine, NYU Winthrop Hospital, Mineola, NY, USA

Jay M. Brenner, MD Department of Emergency Medicine, Upstate Medical University, Syracuse, NY, USA

Arthur R. Derse, MD, JD Center for Bioethics and Medical Humanities, Institute for Health and Equity, and Department of Emergency Medicine, Medical College of Wisconsin, Milwaukee, WI, USA

Holly Fleming, MD Hospital Medicine, Raymond G. Murphy VA Medical Center, Albuquerque, NM, USA

University of New Mexico, Albuquerque, NM, USA

Cynthia Geppert New Mexico Veterans Affairs Health Care System, Department of Psychiatry and Director of Ethics Education, Albuquerque, NM, USA

University of New Mexico School of Medicine, Albuquerque, NM, USA

Alden March Bioethics Institute, Albany Medical College, Albany, NY, USA

Mangla Gulati, MBBS, MD Department of Medicine, University of Maryland School of Medicine, Baltimore, MD, USA

University of Maryland Medical Center, Baltimore, MD, USA

Helen-Maria Lekas, PhD Nathan Kline Institute for Psychiatric Research, Division of Social Solutions and Social Research, Orangeburg, NY, USA

Department of Sociomedical Sciences, Mailman School of Public Health, Columbia University Medical Center, New York, NY, USA

Philip R. Muskin, MD, MA Consultation-Liaison Psychiatry, Columbia University Medical Center, New York, NY, USA

Madhuram Nagarajan, MBBS, MPH Department of Pharmaceutical Health Services Research, University of Maryland School of Pharmacy, Baltimore, MD, USA

Ada Ibe Offurum, MD Department of Medicine, University of Maryland School of Medicine, Baltimore, MD, USA

University of Maryland Medical Center, Baltimore, MD, USA

David S. Olson Jr., MD Department of Internal Medicine, Raymond G. Murphy VA Medical Center, Albuquerque, NM, USA

Eberechukwu Onukwugha, MS, PhD Department of Pharmaceutical Health Services Research, University of Maryland School of Pharmacy, Baltimore, MD, USA

Thomas E. Robey, MD, PhD Elson S. Floyd College of Medicine, Washington State University, Everett, WA, USA

Emergency Department, Providence Regional Medical Center, Everett, WA, USA

North Sound Emergency Medicine, Everett, WA, USA

Jamie L. Shirley, RN, PhD School of Nursing and Health Studies, University of Washington Bothell, Bothell, WA, USA

Part I
Ethical, Legal, and Empirical Considerations

Chapter 1
Introduction

David Alfandre

Introduction

Against medical advice (AMA) discharges occur when a physician formally recognizes a competent patient's choice to decline further inpatient medical care and to leave the hospital prior to a recommended clinical endpoint. Within the USA, these discharges occur frequently, with an established annual prevalence between 1% and 2% of all hospital discharges. Understanding and addressing these discharges are critically important because compared to conventional discharges, AMA discharges are associated with worse health and health service outcomes including higher morbidity, mortality, cost and utilization, and 30-day readmission rate. Patients discharged AMA are a vulnerable population, with disproportionately higher rates of substance use and psychiatric comorbidity and who report stigma and reduced access to care. Caring for these patients has historically been challenging for health-care professionals.

This book serves as a comprehensive resource for a broad audience by consolidating the most up-to-date relevant information and research about AMA discharges in a single volume. By providing a far-reaching examination of AMA discharges and presenting best practices for a multidisciplinary group of health-care professionals, the book can serve as a reference for clinical care, research, and development of professional guidelines and institutional policy.

The views expressed in this article are those of the authors and do not necessarily reflect the position or policy of the U.S. Department of Veterans Affairs, the US Government, or the VA National Center for Ethics in Health Care.

D. Alfandre (✉)
VHA National Center for Ethics in Health Care, Department of Veterans Affairs,
NYU School of Medicine, New York, NY, USA
e-mail: david.alfandre@va.gov

© Springer International Publishing AG, part of Springer Nature 2018
D. Alfandre (ed.), *Against-Medical-Advice Discharges from the Hospital*,
https://doi.org/10.1007/978-3-319-75130-6_1

Throughout the book, the reader will notice a deliberate focus on patient-centered principles as a framework and central solution to the problem of AMA discharges. This decision was motivated by multiple developments in health care as well as its practicality. First is the continuing trend of health systems and professional societies rethinking how their policies and practices can better align with a patient-centered care model. This principle of "patient-centeredness" was driven to prominence when the Institute of Medicine recognized it as essential to quality improvement in health care. In the IOM's 2001 report, *Crossing the Quality Chasm*, they defined patient-centeredness as "providing care that is respectful of and responsive to individual patient preferences, needs, and values and ensuring that patient values guide all clinical decisions." The report was unique not in its determination that quality in health care was defined by the five measures of timeliness, equity, efficiency, effectiveness, and safety but that without the sixth measure of "patient-centeredness" (i.e., that the patient's perspective is a central part of this process), health care would not fulfill its potential.

The chapters throughout this book will return to aforementioned 2001 IOM report and delve deeper into addressing health-care quality in AMA discharges by adapting some of the ten "rules for redesign" described in the IOM report. These rules, more aptly described originally as general principles, were intended to inform system redesign by hewing to the six primary measures of health-care performance described above. The rules are foundational and broad enough to promote strong health practices but still flexible enough to permit local health systems to customize their practices based on their local needs and conditions. The rules for design as applied to improving quality in AMA discharges are briefly described below.

Two of the rules for redesign are directly aligned with patient-centeredness and include "Care is customized according to patient needs and values," and "The patient is the source of control."

These two principles broadly represent the importance of shared decision-making (SDM) and accommodating the range of patient preferences in health-care decisions. SDM enacts patient-centered care by promoting conversations that respect patient's preferences and helps clinicians and patients decide together about a medically acceptable treatment or procedure. In this process, the clinician shares her evidence-based medical knowledge, technical and medical expertise, and experience, and the patient shares his preferences, values, and needs. Armed with this information, the clinician can provide a range of medically acceptable options from which the patient can choose the option that best meets her needs within the context of her life. SDM in discharge planning encourages the patient and provider to work together when there are preference-sensitive (i.e., not value-neutral) decisions to be made about the patient's care. Although this process is typically promoted with value-sensitive decisions when there is more than one reasonable clinical option (e.g., breast or prostate cancer screening) or in end-of-life care, the same process can and should apply to hospital discharge planning. Even though the clinician may initially perceive the range of treatment options to be limited when the patient is hospitalized, there is still a role for identifying when patient's preferences might be relevant to treatment planning and broadening the range of options that could be available.

Care Is Based on Continuous Healing Relationships

This principle promotes care in the many forms and places that patients wish to be treated. Aligning with this principle has led to health-care services provided by email, over the Internet, and telehealth technology in addition to the more traditional face-to-face visits. Applying this principle to the problem of AMA discharges means attempting to accommodate treatment plans to settings outside of the inpatient environment, when medically possible and acceptable, in order to promote continuity of care consistent with the patient's needs and preferences.

Decision-Making Is Evidence-Based

Applying available evidence to the problem of AMA discharges is critical to improving health-care quality. AMA discharges are a routine clinical practice subject to evaluation, and as such, its use should be guided by quality empirical data. At present, the criteria for the determination of an AMA discharge is not standardized and therefore is subject to variability in its use, which is problematic from both a clinical and research perspective. Clinicians counseling patients on the risks, benefits, and alternatives to remaining in the hospital or leaving over their recommendation should base their recommendations on sound empirical data and not primarily on varying clinical opinion.

Transparency Is Necessary

In order for patients to make informed decisions, health-care professionals must disclose all relevant information regarding the risk, benefits and alternatives in discharge planning. Because there are almost always multiple clinical options available for any health-care decision, it is a false choice to provide an option between remaining in the hospital under the conditions specified by the physician and leaving the hospital AMA. Clinical decision-making as part of SDM facilitates transparency by providing patients a range of acceptable medical options, some of which will ideally overlap with their identified needs and preferences.

Needs Are Anticipated

Health-care quality improves when patient's needs are identified early and accurately. The limited data that exists on effective interventions to decrease AMA discharges describes the importance of establishing clear expectations for hospitalized patients. Patients are less likely to leave AMA if clear expectations for treatment are set at the outset of a hospitalization. This information permits patients to have a better sense of the treatment plan and less likely to leave when they believe the plan has changed. This principle is also particularly relevant in patients with opioid use disorders who may wish to leave the hospital to begin using substances again. These patients' clinical needs are better met when inpatient treatment anticipates and delivers medication-assisted treatment (e.g., buprenorphine) for their opioid use disorder. Adequately addressing patients' clinical needs when hospitalized (as well as their relevant personal needs) can facilitate their willingness to complete the inpatient treatment plan.

Cooperation Among Clinicians

The potential for problems with continuity of care are well known when patients are admitted and discharged from the hospital. Although integrated and team-based care is already well established in many health-care systems and is a recognized method to improve quality, the loss of this continuity when seeking inpatient care can distress patients and interfere with hospital-based physician's ability to work productively with patients. Maintaining that connection between inpatient and outpatient providers at both admission and discharge is important in facilitating the trusting bonds needed to promote healing and continuity of care for patients. This may explain in part why patients are more likely to leave AMA when they don't have a primary care provider. Adhering to best practices in transition planning by establishing a clear discharge plan that includes outpatient follow-up with providers known to the patient can facilitate care concordant with the patient's preferences and help to reduce hospital readmission.

Although this book focuses on patient-centered principles for clinical and ethical reasons, it does so for pragmatic reasons as well. For this health-care problem to be adequately addressed, patients must be at the center of workable solutions – no health-care quality problem was ever solved by marginalizing patients. A patient-centered focus works to have the patient's and health-care professional's goals align. AMA discharges unfortunately are defined by their lack of alignment between what the physician recommends and what the patient wants or requests. When these interactions between patients and their health-care providers becomes adversarial as they commonly do, clinicians sometimes focus primarily on their legal liability rather than the care of the patient, and patients focus on their ultimate right to refuse recommended care and exercise any control they have by leaving the hospital. Unfortunately, in that situation, both parties lose. The patient loses a clinician who is engaged and willing to help on the patient's terms, even if suboptimal, and the clinician loses the professional satisfaction of being able to help a patient who needs it.

Health-care practitioners are not simply service providers but rather are dedicated professionals who care for others through their difficult illnesses. To enable these practitioners to develop stable and trusting relationships with patients, they need assistance – we must support the institutions and health-care providers who care for these patients. Preparing health-care professionals to address the AMA discharge problem will require enhanced education at the graduate and postgraduate level, better professional development aimed at patient engagement, professional culture change around sharing power between patients and physicians, and policy and regulatory change to foster clinical practices less centered on legal liability.

In harnessing this patient-centered vision, this book presents itself as a challenge to the long-standing medical model that too often focuses on patients as the sole cause of an AMA discharge and challenges students, trainees, and health-care professionals to reconsider this problem from an alternative perspective. By extending the analysis of this problem beyond the individual patient-physician relationship, we hope to avoid an overly simplistic approach to addressing an otherwise complicated dilemma. Patients are ultimately the ones who choose to leave the hospital setting, but the decision to designate a discharge as AMA is made in a physician-patient relationship with the support of other health-care professionals and administrators, as part of a hospital environment and culture, within an educational and training atmosphere that stresses staff, and amid a larger set of social determinants of patient health that might include poverty and limited access to care. These farther-reaching circumstances that influence AMA discharges are addressed throughout the book by taking a broad lens toward the examination of the AMA problem and toward innovative solutions for redesign of elements of the health-care system.

The book is divided into two separate sections that address the varied aspects of AMA discharges. In the first section, there are six introductory chapters that are written for a wide-ranging audience and provide a broad foundational base with which to understand AMA discharges. These chapters include the ethical, legal, and social science considerations of the problem as well as new perspectives on advancing empirical and normative scholarship and patient-centered clinical practices. Students from all clinical disciplines are likely to find these chapters helpful in better understanding AMA discharges, the problem they pose to the health care system, and how health-care professionals can be meaningful agents of change for better quality. Similarly, all levels of practicing clinicians will find these chapters to be a comprehensive summary but with a renewed patient-centered perspective that extends beyond the traditional characterizations of the issue typically described in the literature.

Chapter 2, "Discharges Against Medical Advice: Prevalence, Predictors, and Populations," provides a comprehensive overview of the existing empirical research on AMA discharges including what populations it occurs in, health-care variables associated with it, and its health and health service outcomes. The analysis examines the hospital, institutional, physician, and social factors beyond the patient that are associated with AMA discharges. This broad perspective on the range of studies devoted to this topic is a jumping-off point for examining the gaps in the literature that highlight the critical need for additional scholarship. Chapter 3, "Legal Considerations of Patient Refusals of Treatment Against Medical Advice," provides a practical overview of the legal aspects of working with patients who decline recommended care. Although the current literature in this area is sparse, anecdotal reports and expert opinion suggest that the legal landscape of this problem, including institutional and individual liability, significantly influences health-care professionals' thought process and behavior. The chapter describes the legal requirements for informed consent in discharge planning, the relevance of decision-making capacity, and a description of the use of AMA discharge forms in managing individual and institutional liability. This legal analysis provides needed grounding for addressing the related ethical and clinical issues throughout the remainder of the book. In Chap. 4, "Ethical Considerations in Against Medical Advice Discharges: Values Conflicts over Patient Autonomy and Best Interests," the authors review the major ethical principles that apply to the effective management of AMA discharges. By focusing on the principles of respect for autonomy, shared decision-making, and harm reduction, this chapter provides a normative basis for the recommendations made throughout the book and will assist clinicians and educators in promoting these grounding principles more transparently to colleagues, students, and trainees. Chapter 5, "Reframing the Phenomenon of Discharges Against Medical Advice: A Sociologist's Perspective," expands upon the existing medical model of AMA discharges with a social science perspective and an analysis of the social roles that physicians, patients, and health-care institutions play in AMA discharges. Through this perspective, we can discern the mechanisms operating on the individual, interpersonal, institutional, and social levels that undermine the provision of patient-centered care and may contribute to health disparities. This chapter represents a new and emerging direction in AMA discharges research by using qualitative data from health records and physician and patient interviews to provide new solutions to address the frequent communication problems seen with AMA discharges. Chapter 6, "Social Justice and the Ethics of Care: A Nursing Perspective," explores the problem of AMA discharges from the vantage point of promoting equitable access to health care and the critical role that therapeutic relationships play in doing so. The author provides practical guidance for achieving these goals, by appreciating patients' social context, committing to creative action in problem-solving, interprofessional collaboration, and attending to care transitions.

Because AMA discharges are not just a quality problem, but a discrete clinical problem that occurs in all fields of inpatient medicine, the second section of the book is divided into relevant medical specialty in order to address the context-specific aspects of the problem. Chapters specific to AMA discharges in the emergency department, pediatric, and psychiatric settings have been provided to give those practicing clinicians up-to-date high-quality information that will inform their practice. Chapter 7, "Bedside Management of Discharges Against Medical Advice," reviews the current best practices, interventions, and communication strategies to address requests to leave the hospital over the recommendation of the physician. Clinicians will appreciate the specific tools, heuristics, and conceptual grounding that will guide practitioners in managing these complicated clinical and ethical dilemmas. This chapter, which is written for practicing clinicians and educators, will also help teach these skills to health-care professional trainees as part of daily hospital care and contemporaneously when the issue presents itself with a patient.

Chapter 8, "Against Medical Advice Discharges from the Emergency Department," provides a comprehensive analysis of the problem from the perspective of emergency providers. The unique demands and challenges of working with patients in the emergency department means that specific knowledge and skill sets are needed to adequately care for patients who choose to leave AMA from this care setting. Because many patients discharged AMA have co-occurring psychiatric disorders, substance use disorders, and counterproductive reactions to the hospital environment, Chap. 9, "To Thy Own Self Be True: Contributions from Consultation-Liaison Psychiatry," was written to provide physicians with specific management skills as well as communication strategies for patients wishing to leave over the recommendation of their health-care provider. In Chap. 10, "Against Medical Advice Discharges: Pediatric Considerations," there is a review of the topic as it applies to pediatric patients, including how to effectively frame challenging discharge discussions with parents, relevant legal considerations unique to that population, and maintaining the therapeutic alliance with patients and their parents when there is disagreement. Chapter 11, "Against Medical Advice Discharges: Considerations in the Psychiatric Population," includes guidance for the practicing psychiatrist regarding declination of inpatient psychiatric care. Because there are unique ethical and legal considerations in hospitalized patients with mental health illnesses, the chapter will examine specific issues to this population including criteria for commitment and discharge planning in vulnerable populations.

This book is the first comprehensive examination of the problem of AMA discharges in medicine and hopefully will not be its last. Students, trainees, faculty, administrators, quality managers, health service researchers, and clinicians need guidance in conceptualizing and addressing this problem now and for the future. Now is the time to tackle this problem in new and innovative ways. We hope that this book helps to educate, inspire, advance scholarship, and begin to close some of the quality gaps around AMA discharges. Finally, we hope that this publication forges a path forward that engages health-care professionals, improves health-care quality, is patient-centered, and helps to promote care that recognizes and respects patient's preferences and desire to participate in important health-care decisions.

Suggested Reading

1. Alfandre DJ. "I'm going home": discharges against medical advice. Mayo Clin Proc. 2009;84(3):255–60.
2. Alfandre D. Reconsidering against medical advice discharges: embracing patient-centeredness to promote high quality care and a renewed research agenda. J Gen Intern Med. 2013;28(12):1657–62.
3. Institute of Medicine (US). Committee on Quality of Health Care in America. Crossing the quality chasm: a new health system for the 21st century. Washington, DC: National Academy Press; 2001.

Chapter 2
Discharges Against Medical Advice: Prevalence, Predictors, and Populations

Madhuram Nagarajan, Ada Ibe Offurum, Mangla Gulati, and Eberechukwu Onukwugha

Introduction

Discharge against medical advice (DAMA) is defined as when a patient leaves a healthcare institution, typically a hospital, before the recommendation of the treating physician [1]. This is also called against medical advice (AMA), or leaving against medical advice (LAMA), and may be referred to colloquially as a patient "absconding." DAMA is an understudied problem that leads to worse patient outcomes, and there are significant gaps in what has been studied in the literature.

In the United States (USA), DAMA constitutes 1–2% of all hospital discharges annually [2–4] or approximately 500,000 discharges annually [5, 6]. A number of studies examined outcomes following an AMA discharge [2–5] and found a higher likelihood of 30-day readmission (hazard ratio = 1.35 [2]; hazard ratio = 2.5 [3]). In one study, DAMA increased the likelihood of readmission by 21% in the first 15 days [3]. Patients leaving AMA also had a higher 30-day mortality rate compared to the remainder of the discharge population (0.75% vs 0.61%), even after controlling for patient demographics and comorbidities [2]. Patients who leave AMA may be reluctant to return to the hospital despite having ongoing or recurrent symptoms or needing further evaluation [7].

Research to date has centered primarily on patient-related factors, including who might be considered a high-risk patient for DAMA [2, 5, 8], and on how to discuss options with (and document) a patient wanting to leave AMA [9, 10]. It may be the

M. Nagarajan · E. Onukwugha (✉)
Department of Pharmaceutical Health Services Research, University of Maryland School of Pharmacy, Baltimore, MD 21201, USA
e-mail: eonukwug@rx.umaryland.edu

A. I. Offurum · M. Gulati
Department of Medicine, University of Maryland School of Medicine, Baltimore, MD 21201, USA

University of Maryland Medical Center, Baltimore, MD 21201, USA

© Springer International Publishing AG, part of Springer Nature 2018
D. Alfandre (ed.), *Against-Medical-Advice Discharges from the Hospital*,
https://doi.org/10.1007/978-3-319-75130-6_2

11

case that at the point when the patient indicates that they wish to leave the hospital, it is too late to prevent the DAMA. In order to target avoidable DAMA, clinicians need evidence-based interventions and risk-reduction measures that are delivered in a timely fashion. The development of effective interventions depends on a rich evidence base to identify the contributing factors, not all of which will be patient-level factors.

In this book chapter, we synthesize the existing literature on DAMA and provide a framework to consider what is known or has been reported to date. The framework provides a common basis from which to describe the contributing factors, identify areas for further research, and consider what types of interventions can be developed to reduce preventable DAMA and the consequent negative outcomes for the patient, provider, and healthcare system. The book chapter is divided into three sections. In the first section, we introduce our conceptual framework within the context of a scoping literature review. We then discuss the findings from the literature review and describe its public health significance. The final section considers next steps for research on DAMA based on actionable levers to improve patient health outcomes associated with a DAMA.

Literature Review

Methods

We conducted multiple searches with two independent reviewers, using PubMed, Embase, Scopus, and Web of Science. Both team members used these keywords, "against medical advice," "discharge against medical advice," "AMA," "DAMA," "patient discharge," and "risk factors," in various combinations and with upper and lower case variations and searched in the title and abstract of published papers for these keywords. There was no single MeSH term or equivalent that encompassed this category that we could find in our searches. We limited our search to items published on or after January 1, 2000, with exceptions made for key articles that were repeatedly cited and for our historic lookback in the search engines. We conducted the literature review over a period of 3 months. All authors contributed to this phase of the project by providing input on the design of the literature review (e.g., data parameters, target populations), forwarding key articles, or suggesting key words to use in the review. We focused our review on the adult general inpatient population to make our discussion broad and generalizable. In the review process, we encountered a number of articles on populations with special considerations. We discuss these populations briefly in a subsection that follows.

We restricted our review to studies that reported on patients residing in the United States. We made exceptions regarding specific articles from Canada or Australia that offered generalizable findings with no equivalent study conducted in the United States. Although we restricted our literature review to the US setting, we took care to address general and globally applicable issues in our conceptual framework. We reviewed relevant individual articles on the list and eliminated those that either were not relevant to the topic or that did not meet the criteria discussed above. We conducted a backward search in order to manually identify more articles and achieve saturation on this topic.

Conceptual Framework

Our review of the articles in our defined search on DAMA identified several themes and causal threads across this literature. The studies could be broadly categorized into two groups: one group consisted of retrospective, quantitative observational studies based on a large population of hospital discharges. These studies reported factors that were associated with a DAMA. The second group of studies utilized qualitative research methods – interviews, focus groups – and, as such, involved a smaller number of patients. These studies reported the patients' reasons for leaving the hospital AMA from patient and clinical provider perspectives. We divided the list of factors into two columns, each to represent one of these groups (Table 2.1). In the table, we reference the studies by each individual factor. The first column focuses on quantifiable factors associated with increased likelihood of DAMA, while the second qualitative column helps to understand the situation proximate to the decision to leave AMA. We believe that both groups of studies have their roles to play in helping us understand the complex reasons for DAMA and in designing effective interventions.

In our review, we found that many of the issues that influence a patient's reported decision to leave AMA are independent of the patient's characteristics. For this reason, we divided Table 2.1 into patient-level and non-patient-level factors related to DAMA. We created the conceptual framework in Fig. 2.1 to organize the various factors related to DAMA and refined it further through our internal discussions from the clinical and health service research perspectives. In creating the framework, we drew from the literature on the socioecological model of human development and health education [11, 12].

The framework has, at the center, the individual and the individual-level factors. This innermost circle consists of the characteristics of the individual or of their health status. For instance, characteristics of the individual include age, gender, race, socioeconomic status, education, and employment – some of these are mutable, while others are not. The individual's health status could feature behaviors such as exercise, diet, tobacco and alcohol consumption, sexual behavior, religious beliefs, as well as illnesses.

In concentric circles around the individual-level factors are the factors at the interpersonal level, the community level, and the societal level. The interpersonal level is conceptualized as the proximate contacts that the individual has with the broader society and can vary based on context. For most people, this consists of their partner, relationships with family or extended family, a network of friends, colleagues from work, and acquaintances from leisure activities. In the context of

Table 2.1 Quantitative factors and qualitative factors in discharge against medical advice from a review of the literature

Factors related to AMA	Quantitative factors	Qualitative factors
Patient level	Demographics:	Treatment related:
	Male [2, 4, 5, 8, 13, 14]	Felt better [4, 15, 16]
	Younger age [2, 4, 5, 8, 13, 14]	Unhappy with care received [4]
	African-American [2, 4, 5, 13]	Perception of disrespect or unfair treatment [17]
	Hispanic (lower) [5, 13]	Not involved in decision-making [16]
	Socioeconomic status:	Substance use related:
	Income [2, 4]	Drug addiction or drug-seeking [17]
	Lower education levels [4]	Poor management of drug withdrawal [15, 18]
	Access to care:	Poor in-hospital pain management [17]
	Individuals with Medicare, Medicaid, or self-pay [4, 5, 8, 13, 14]	External drivers:
	No personal physician (primary care physician) [13, 15]	Family concerns/obligations [4, 17, 19]
	Preexisting disease states:	Work/financial related [4, 15, 17]
	Mental health disorders [5]	Patient preference:
		Preference for their own physician [16]
	Substance abuse-related disorders [13]	Personal reasons [4, 15]
	Cancer related (lower) [5]	
	Greater comorbidities (lower) [5, 8]	
	Healthcare resource utilization related:	
	Admission from the ER [4, 8, 13]	
	Increasing length of stay(lower) [4, 5]	
	Previous AMA discharge [15]	
Non-patient level	Hospital related:	Communication related:
	Medium or large hospitals [5, 14]	Poor communication between providers
	Teaching hospitals (lower) [5, 14]	Poor communication with the patient [16, 17]
	Not-for-profit hospitals (lower) [8]	Patient not clearly told about risks of DAMA [18]
	Extremes of concentration of hospital ownership (HHI) [8]	Poor relationship with the community being served by the hospital
	Geography related:	Treatment related:
	Urban [5, 8, 14]	Inadequate pain management [16]
	Low median income of the patient's ZIP code of residence [5, 8]	Administrative or other delays:
		Delays in testing, treatment, or discharge
	Northeast region [14]	Process [16, 17]
		Delay in discharge because of patient age or physician inexperience

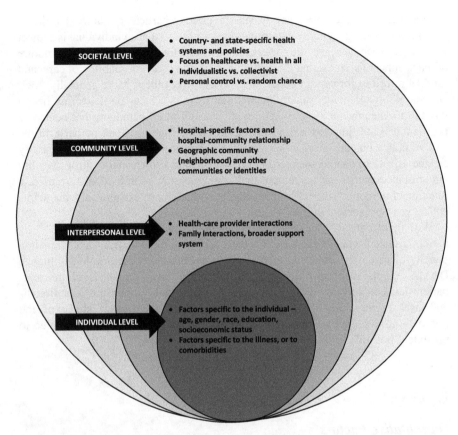

Fig. 2.1 A framework for considering the various dimensions of a decision to leave against medical advice [11, 12]

healthcare, it consists of their primary care provider, if they have one; if they are admitted into a hospital or nursing facility, it includes their relationship with the physicians, nurses, and other providers who care for them during their stay, communication with their healthcare providers, and perceptions of being respected and given high-quality care.

The community level includes the geographic community that an individual lives in and works but also encompasses various identities and associations that the person forms – cultural, religious, political, professional, or social labels a person may have or, more formally, organizations that a person may belong to. It also includes the hospital or health system that an individual has been admitted to, the perception of the hospital in the community (or communities) that the person belongs to, and relations between the hospital and the community.

The societal level can be conceived of as the overarching social environment that the individual lives, works, and obtains healthcare services in. It is in one sense geographic, such as a particular city, state, region, or particular country; but this is only insofar as the geography determines the conditions that an individual is subject to. In a very specific sense, the society an individual lives in influences the structure of the healthcare systems that are available, access to care, affordability of care, and funding priorities for certain goods and services over others. More generally, societal and political choices determine whether there is a focus on delivering health through the healthcare system or through a health-in-all paradigm that considers population health impacts when making all policy (more visible, perhaps, in the case of policy on education, employment, and housing). More difficult to quantify are the effects of shared societal beliefs with regard to personal control over life circumstances versus an agreement that some measure of individual fortune is a function of random chance at birth or that individual liberty is more valuable than a collective improvement of the whole.

With this framework and these levels in mind, dividing the list in Table 2.1 by patient and non-patient factors served to reinforce our position that there is a paucity of research dealing with the non-individual-level factors that influence DAMA. We have chosen, therefore, to divide the list in patient-level and non-patient-level factors, by aggregating the interpersonal-, community-, and societal-level factors; we are cognizant of the need for further study of the non-patient-level factors so that these levels and factors may be disentangled to the extent possible from one another.

Results

Quantitative Factors

These patient-level factors for DAMA are well known and have been included in multiple studies. Some of the factors associated with an increased likelihood for leaving AMA include male gender, younger age, African-American race, individuals without insurance or with Medicare or Medicaid coverage, mental illness, and substance use disorders including alcohol abuse [3–5, 8, 13].

However, there are non-patient-level factors that are associated with an increased odds of leaving AMA – these include the setting of the hospital (with urban hospitals having increased odds), the size of the hospital (with medium and to a lesser extent large hospitals having increased odds), the type of hospital (with teaching hospitals and nonprofit hospitals having a lower odds), and the route of admission (with admission through the emergency room conferring a higher odds) [5, 8, 13].

There are certain non-patient-level factors that are difficult to measure that may contribute to different rates of DAMA and nonetheless bear investigating. These include provider communication quality, which has been quantified in other research questions, access to and availability of outpatient health service, and hospital organizational factors that lead to administrative delays in discharge.

The Patient Needing Hemodialysis

Mr. H, a 26-year-old male with no medical insurance, was admitted for kidney failure in the setting of untreated hypertension. The nephrology team had to determine whether his kidneys would be able to recover function or not for which the patient remained in the hospital for 3 weeks with close monitoring of his electrolytes and fluid status. During this time, he expressed his desire to take care of his home and ensure his daughter (who was in the care of his mother) was doing well. He was told to be patient, and he was.

After he was transitioned to a regular dialysis schedule, it was a challenge to find him an outpatient dialysis facility because he lacked any form of insurance. After waiting an additional week for the case manager/social worker to find a community dialysis center, he left AMA.

Certain factors may have effects that are not apparent at the level of the individual patient or within a hospital but can be seen in differential outcomes at the population level. DAMA may well be an outcome of this kind because minority status and socioeconomic status, insurance status, and admission in large, urban, teaching hospitals may show significant correlation [8]. There is an interaction between race and patient perception of high-quality care [20], which may extend to other measures that have not been examined. We discuss these multilevel factors and how their effects may be disentangled and better understood in the section on Public Health Significance.

Qualitative (Precipitating) Factors

The focus of the qualitative studies on DAMA has been to get answers to the vexing question "Given the risks to the patient's health, why did the patient choose to leave AMA?" Although the factors discussed above chiefly focused on patient characteristics associated with DAMA, when patients are asked about their leaving, they identified reasons related to circumstances outside the patient's control as often as their own, personal desire to leave [5, 8, 13, 16].

From Table 2.1, we see that the reasons given by patients can be categorized as treatment-related concerns, such as a perception that they are not given respect or good care; substance abuse-related reasons, such as inadequate pain management and lack of support for drug withdrawal; external drivers such as taking care of family or work; and personal preferences.

The Patient with Sickle Cell Disease

Ms. V, a 22-year-old with sickle cell disease, had recently moved to New York from Virginia, where she attended college. While in college, she had a good relationship with her hematology outpatient group. Her illness often required admission once every 3 months for a vaso-occlusive crisis that caused acute pain, and she was cared for in the pediatric ward of a teaching hospital. She was close to the providers on the ward, and she appreciated when they had a farewell party on her graduation from college.

During her present admission on an adult inpatient unit in New York, the patient cried while discussing her prior experiences in Virginia compared to the treatment she was receiving in New York. She described repeated crises during her short time in New York. When she asked for pain medications during these episodes, she was told that the providers did not want to support opioid dependence. She felt like she had moved to a place with a different attitude toward patients with sickle cell disease and where her pain was poorly managed. She left the hospital AMA because she believed that going back to her previous care providers would help her condition and that if she did not go back, her illness would worsen and she would be left with long-term complications.

The non-patient-level factors listed in the table are, to a large extent, a function of circumstances and the support system available to the patient – the need to care for a loved one, not being able to get a ride, patients not wanting to wait for administrative delays, work obligations that could not be put off, and frustration with the process of healthcare delivery.

Special Populations

The literature review focused on the general medical inpatient population, but in the process we identified a number of articles focusing on special populations. We excluded them in our general discussion but will briefly discuss unique considerations in certain vulnerable patient populations, such as in patients with psychiatric disorders or substance use disorders, pediatric patients, obstetrics and gynecology (OB/GYN) patients, and patients with linguistic barriers.

The psychiatric population has among the higher prevalence rates of DAMA with estimates ranging from 3% to 51%, with a mean of 17% [21]. One of the chief considerations in the psychiatric population when discussing DAMA is the question of decision-making capacity (DMC) to choose to leave inpatient care. DMC is not only the strict capacity to understand what is being conveyed but more broadly a capacity to understand their medical condition and appreciate the potential consequences of discharge AMA. Factors for psychiatric patients leaving AMA were similar to the general population and included young age, male gender, comorbid substance use, previous discharge AMA, and provider variables such as a failure to orient patients to their surroundings. Specific factors in the psychiatric population included greater severity of psychiatric illness at diagnosis, patients not taking medication, behavioral factors, and a pessimistic attitude toward treatment [21, 22].

In DAMA in the pediatric population, the chief consideration is that children do not make the decision to leave AMA for themselves – their parent or guardian is often the decision-maker. Hence there is a greater need for communication to ensure the caregiver understands the care plan and documentation if they decide to leave AMA. Patients in this population were more likely to leave AMA if they were in the age group of 15–20 years of age, came by ambulance to the ER, and admitted themselves (unaccompanied by parents) [23]. Other reasons were if the parent thinks the child is well, financial constraints, time lost from work, and dissatisfaction with treatment [24].

The obstetric population is a special group because of the vulnerability of the fetus in utero to medical conditions affecting the mother. Discharge AMA can be divided into antepartum and postpartum groups. Factors associated with increased likelihood of leaving AMA antepartum included African-American race, public insurance, and mental illness or substance use [25]. Leaving AMA antepartum was associated with 3 times the odds of fetal death, 1.3 times the odds of neonatal respiratory distress syndrome, and 1.47 times the odds of being small for gestational age [25]. Given the small number of studies and the significant risk to human health, this population needs further study and characterization. The postpartum population had an average DAMA rate of 0.10% [26], and associated factors were similar to antepartum DAMA. The rates of leaving AMA were lowest in women with uncomplicated deliveries, intermediate in complicated vaginal deliveries, and highest following complicated C-sections [26]. Because these patients have an increased likelihood of readmission to hospital, they may benefit from the delivery of targeted services [26].

We also considered patients who face linguistic, religious, and cultural barriers to be a population that requires further characterization. We discuss them in this paragraph as a group, even though they are quite heterogeneous, due to common barriers in understanding their medical condition, communicating their wishes to healthcare providers, and participating fully in decision-making on their care. A medical translator is particularly helpful in these circumstances. These patients may also not want to be documented in the system, and their concerns over not having residency or citizenship documentation raise the threshold to seek medical care and make this population reluctant to remain in the hospital. These patients may also have concerns about insurance and payment of medical bills that need to be addressed in order to ensure that they remain in hospital to receive medically necessary care.

Public Health Significance

Discharge against medical advice is a substantial burden, and the rate of leaving AMA appears to be rising with a 1.9% average annual increase in its prevalence each year between 2002 and 2011 [14]. As we have seen, patients who leave AMA are likely to be sicker when they return and are reluctant to return despite having symptoms [7]. The associated factors, including the personal characteristics of those more likely to leave AMA [2, 4, 5, 13], predispose them to worse health and health services outcomes and to experience societal and economic disadvantages; in addition, they are more likely to be distrustful of the health system and have obligations to return to [4, 17, 19]. This suggests a greater public health focus on the numbers of patients who leave AMA and how we can address this issue. We also know that DAMA leads to poorer outcomes in the form of increased 30-day readmission [3] and increased 30-day mortality [2] and greater health expenditure than if the patient had remained in the hospital and completed treatment [27]. All this points to a need for a greater focus on the numbers of patients who leave AMA and how we can address this issue.

The problem of DAMA has typically been framed as one of individual patient choices. From that perspective, the patient is a rational actor and chooses to leave AMA after considering all the information available and after considering their own overall desires and maximal benefit [28]. From this perspective, health is not an ultimate good or even the only good – leisure, work, and other considerations may all trump the utility of seeking healthcare at a given point [28, 29]. If we were to consider this matter as a specific individual in certain circumstances leaving AMA, it may seem to be a unique combination of factors that can be "explained" after a fashion – and frequently, that "explanation" may be met with disapproval by healthcare providers [16, 19]. However, when we view this decision from the population health perspective, we see the commonalities between the various individual "explanations" and might begin to appreciate why individuals make certain choices.

We know from work in behavioral economics that individuals are not purely rational actors – whether they are seeking healthcare [30], providing healthcare [31], or making decisions with regard to who obtains healthcare, at whose cost, and of what quality. These behavioral factors also condition how patients perceive the risk of illness [32–35], the kind of care-seeking behavior they exhibit [30], and their level of trust in the system [36]. For instance, a vividly described but extremely rare adverse reaction to a vaccine may be perceived as more risky and commonly occurring than the consequences of not being vaccinated and getting the illness [35]. Absolute numbers seem to be better understood by people than proportions or percentages [32] – hence the memorable title of a paper by Yamagishi et al., "When a 12.86% mortality is more dangerous than 24.14%," which described how "participants rated cancer as riskier when it was described as 'kills 1,286 out of 10,000 people' than as 'kills 24.14 out of 100 people'."

We also recognize that individuals do not exist in splendid solitude, isolated from social, religious, cultural, and political systems. For instance, at the interpersonal level, interactions with healthcare providers and the hospital system have a role to play in patients' decisions to leave AMA. While race may be an individual characteristic, it also is affected by how that element of patient identity interacts more broadly with provider attitudes and communication [37] and with the larger society the individual lives in [38]. The influence of the broader community, in terms of trust of the hospital system and healthcare providers, availability and accessibility of services in certain communities, and availability of support systems – all these can affect the likelihood of a patient remaining in the hospital versus leaving AMA. A final influence is the effect of even broader societal decisions on individuals making choices to leave AMA. These include policies regarding insurance coverage, tax distribution toward community services, resources allocated to population health measures, and health insurance models (e.g., fee-for-service models) and whether DAMA events are enumerated and viewed as a measure of quality of care.

We submit that there are real dangers to viewing DAMA as a "problem" with a specific set of patients – perhaps even considering them "problem patients" – because it centers the problem on the patients and their choices without due consideration of the broader influences. Patients labeled in this manner using terms such as noncompliant may be viewed by the healthcare system and by providers as disagreeable or even foolish in refusing to listen to medical advice. A record that the patient has been previously DAMA in the chart may color present and future interactions with healthcare providers and perpetuate dysfunctional therapeutic relationships and a distrust of the system on the part of the patient [15, 17]. At base, it undermines the notion of autonomy and patient-centered healthcare [39, 40] and endangers patients who may be discharged without prescriptions or follow-up instructions [10, 40, 41].

For healthcare providers, there are chances that a "problem" patient's complaints may be perceived as being less serious or a patient's narrative of their illness, veracity, and adherence to medication being doubted [9, 31]. Using an individual-choice paradigm for DAMA also leads to a sense of helplessness on the part of the provider – "It's inexplicable, but it's what the patient wants and nothing can be done about it"; if anything, multiple studies have shown that patients leaving AMA remain open to physician follow-up on the phone, medications, and instructions [15, 16]. Healthcare providers should recognize that they still retain their capacity to advise and influence even when patients are leaving AMA. Assessment of decision-making capacity, and if a patient truly understands what their discharge might mean, is important, and conflict de-escalation and motivational interviewing are skills that can be learned and used. One observation stood out over the course of our review; that discussions of how healthcare providers might deal with patients choosing DAMA begin and end with an exhortation to document that the patient is leaving AMA [9]. Physicians need to recognize that a signature on a DAMA form is not a waiver of liability [42]. There is still a need to assess and document patient competency and understanding of their medical condition and to provide as much medical care as the patient will accept [41].

In addition, there is a commonly held misperception among physicians that leaving AMA can result in the insurer refusing to cover the cost of the patient's stay

[43]. This is inaccurate at best, and well-intentioned mention of this to patients and their families may leave them feeling coerced to stay in the hospital, further straining the provider-patient relationship. Paradoxically, physicians admitting patients for "observation" because of readmission incentives to the hospital system [44] may lead to patients leaving earlier than medically recommended due to cost. CMS considers observation status an outpatient service under Medicare policy, and Medicare Part B services have a deductible amount that the patient is responsible for. In addition, the patient ends up bearing 20% of the cost of their stay across all services provided [45, 46], leaving them with a hefty out-of-pocket payment. In line with CMS, many private insurers have a lower reimbursement rate for observation status, again resulting in greater out-of-pocket costs for patients [45].

Another situation where the patient may be left bearing the costs of hospitalization is when the patient has been admitted even though the insurer's stringent criteria of medical necessity for admission or observation [45, 46] may not have been met. This may arise from clinical judgment or because of the patient's living situation (typically someone who is elderly, living alone, living in a remote area, or not having access to personal transport). In these cases as well, their stay will not be covered by insurance. In both these situations, admission or observation status decisions are made by the admitting physician, and it is important for physicians to be aware of the cost issues and be transparent with the patient regarding their stay status, planned length of stay, and cost implications for the patient.

The biggest problem with accepting that patient-level factors alone are key with regard to DAMA is the lost opportunity to better examine and evaluate the underlying structural issues that may contribute to and perpetuate the problem. If we accept that some patients just leave AMA without closely examining and addressing the reasons, the same patterns will repeat themselves. We need to shift the discussion around DAMA from being an intractable problem focused on patients to being, instead, a manageable problem with research being conducted on broader, non-patient-level factors and specific interventions to assess impact on the problem.

Directions for Future Research

There is a great deal left to be characterized and understood about the impact of non-patient-level factors on the decision to leave AMA. The framework we have proposed in Fig. 2.1 is a useful tool to classify factors that might influence DAMA and also to consider what cluster of interventions at various levels might shift this outcome, keeping in mind that groups of interventions at different levels might have a greater impact than a single intervention that addresses one level of this model.

At the patient level, we might consider more holistic discharge planning involving patients early in the admission. It may be the case that at the point when the patient brings up that they wish to leave the hospital, it is too late to prevent the DAMA. Interventions and risk-reduction measures need to be delivered before the situation escalates to the point of a DAMA. We could also change the narrative of

DAMA as being a rejection of all medical care, instead reframing it as a choice to accept some services but not others. We can continue to monitor these patients who have chosen to leave AMA, perhaps by calling and following up – something that focus groups have indicated might be well received [16].

There has been some study of provider characteristics (such as communication styles) and patient outcomes (and satisfaction), but not much work done on the impact provider characteristics might have on DAMA. An intervention that hospitals might consider is adding DAMA to the physician scorecard. It might be helpful to do a root cause analysis with the care team when a patient leaves AMA and to discuss these at routine clinical meetings such as morbidity and mortality rounds.

There is limited information available about hospital-level characteristics that may contribute to DAMA. The study of the influence of hospital characteristics on DAMA requires researchers to be able to look at large, nationally representative datasets offering linkages to other datasets with hospital characteristics. For instance, a particularly intriguing associated factor that came up in our literature review was that hospital concentration at extremes was associated with DAMA, measured using the Herfindahl-Henderson Index (HHI), a measure of market concentration. This is timely since there has been increasing consolidation of hospitals and physician practices since this paper came out in 2006 [8] to where we are now in 2017, and simultaneous rates of DAMA have been increasing nationally [14]. There is a great deal of work to be done to understand associations between hospital and community characteristics and DAMA.

One avenue for hospital-level intervention is using measurement to ensure our health system starts counting and caring for this patient population. We know that the count of patients being discharged AMA is substantial, estimated to be roughly 500,000 every year [5, 6]; the average annual period prevalence appears to have been increasing over the period of 2002–2011 [14]. There is limited research focused on identifying interventions to reduce the rates of patients leaving care before it is considered medically appropriate. In this data void, we propose that collecting this information in a systematic manner across the US health system on rates of DAMA is the bare minimum needed to understand and begin to design interventions for DAMA.

Standardized data collection on DAMA requires us to agree on what is considered DAMA and apply a standard set of protocols if patients indicate a desire to be discharged AMA. For instance, there are varying sets of forms used for discharge by different institutions – some use a regular discharge form while documenting that the patient wishes to leave AMA, others have a special form for DAMA, and in some instances patients may be discharged without forms or follow-up. There is little agreement on what constitutes DAMA or what is to be documented in the chart with regard to the patient's decision-making capacity to leave AMA, the patient's understanding of the potential implications of discharge AMA, and the patient's willingness to take medications and follow instructions regarding care [41]. In some instances, DAMA may not be documented in the chart because the provider did not wish to "put a blemish on the patient's record" [4].

Another avenue for intervention is that at present, there is no underlying administrative requirement for reporting data on DAMA, standardization of data collection, or examination of quality improvement indicators of DAMA (with financial penalties attached) – we do not even require a basic prevalence of DAMA to be reported by hospitals. Indicators of DAMA are not rolled into other measures of hospital performance either; in fact, patients who leave AMA are excluded from the count and formula used to calculate 30-day readmissions by the Centers for Medicare and Medicaid Services (CMS) [47, 48]. The rationale given is that with patients who leave AMA, the hospital has not had a sufficient opportunity to intervene in the patient's health [47]; hence this population should not impact hospital's numbers and subsequent reimbursement by CMS. The idea of "insufficient opportunity to intervene" is not only a dated notion when managing population health is a priority but removes the responsibility for DAMA from the providers and the hospital system. By not counting these patients, CMS, covering 57 million on Medicare [49] and 75 million enrolled on Medicaid [50], may be missing an opportunity to influence the quality of provider communication and to encourage holistic discharge planning.

We mentioned the numbers of DAMA annually being comparable to 30-day readmissions and the efforts put in by hospitals to control the latter in order to highlight the impact of CMS reimbursement and penalty policies. Readmissions are expensive, and it would seem that lowering readmission rates ought to mean better patient care and less expensive medical care. Yet there are issues with whether readmissions truly reflect hospital quality, the burden of reporting, diverting time and effort from other quality improvement initiatives, and that perhaps only 27% [51, 52] of readmissions were truly preventable. The hospitals that received the greatest burden of penalties with the Hospital Readmissions Reduction Program (HRRP) were urban, large, teaching hospitals that served a population with greater proportions of Medicare or low SES patients [53], and some of these factors not captured by the case-mix ratio may explain the variation in hospital readmission rate [53]. Socioeconomic and demographic factors play a large role in health indicators, including readmission rates [53] and DAMA [51]. Many hospitals receive penalties year after year which might impact their ability to invest in readmission reduction measures [54].

Readmission measures offer us useful lessons we might apply to any future incentives or penalties we might consider for DAMA – lessons in how incentives and penalties may need to be structured to avoid "gaming" of the system (for instance, by admitting under observation status) [44] as well as other unintended consequences such as penalizing hospitals serving poorer, sicker populations. If we are to move in the direction of tracking DAMA, we would need to consider robust DAMA-specific measures and design policy to avoid hospitals falling into a DAMA-penalty trap, as is happening with readmission measures at this time.

We believe that we can study how features of health systems and health policy, the overarching level within which patient interactions are embedded, can be tweaked to benefit patient care and reduce rates of DAMA. A policy-level intervention we might consider is incentivizing accountable care organizations that manage populations, where it is in the health system's interests to make available outpatient resources so patients are not admitted to the hospital to access care that is available in the outpatient setting. This might take the form of stronger support systems and care coordination to ensure that people who need to remain in hospital can do so rather than leave prematurely to meet obligations and get readmitted with complications.

An area of inquiry we might consider is comparative health system study, examining the characteristics of other health systems and policies and seeing how they might apply to our specific context and populations. It was evident from our review that DAMA is a topic that is of interest across countries, and we believe that there is a place for future research that compares across health systems and societies.

The increase in the number of publications on DAMA from 1998 [13] onward [2–5, 8, 17, 18, 23, 39] is heartening, and there is a greater awareness of and interest in understanding this challenge at present [9, 14]. We intended for our review to highlight the lacunae in our present understanding of DAMA and that our framework helps set the direction of future research into contributing causal factors at the different levels and to the design of interventions. A good start might be checklists put in standardized intake and discharge forms to identify patients as being at risk for DAMA, analogous to fall risk or pressure ulcer risk. Another place to begin attacking DAMA rates would be designing multilevel interventions using the information we already have and to test these measures in pilot studies, followed by implementation at scale. However, these kinds of measures would require a commitment from providers, hospitals, and framers of health policy.

What happens now? In our review, one of the earliest articles we found was in relation to the "irregular discharge of tuberculous patients" [55], from a time when patients were still being admitted and advised months of bedrest for treatment of tuberculosis with only limited effective pharmacologic options [56]. Patients might have been understandably skeptical about the possibility of a cure and were tired of being confined to bed. We might be able to offer definitive treatments for a broader spectrum of illness, but we are in a similar place when we consider "treatments" for DAMA. As we look ahead, will we merely produce confirmatory findings [15, 55, 57–63], or will we identify effective interventions? We do not know at this time what proportion of DAMA is preventable and how much of it is due to factors outside the control of patients, providers and hospitals. We do know, however, that our collective societal response to this vulnerable, poorly served population will be telling.

References

1. Venes D, Taber CW. Taber's cyclopedic medical dictionary. Philadelphia: F.A. Davis Co.; 2013.; 2013. Available from: http://survey.hshsl.umaryland.edu/?url=http://search.ebscohost.com/login.aspx?direct=true&db=cat01362a&AN=hshs.004293179&site=eds-live.
2. Glasgow JM, Vaughn-Sarrazin M, Kaboli PJ. Leaving against medical advice (AMA): risk of 30-day mortality and hospital readmission. J Gen Intern Med. 2010;25(9):926–9.

3. Hwang SW, Li J, Gupta R, Chien V, Martin RE. What happens to patients who leave hospital against medical advice? CMAJ 2003 Feb 18 [cited 2017 Jan 5];168(4):417–20. Available from: http://www.ncbi.nlm.nih.gov/pubmed/12591781.
4. Baptist AP, Warrier I, Arora R, Ager J, Massanari RM. Hospitalized patients with asthma who leave against medical advice: characteristics, reasons, and outcomes. J Allergy Clin Immunol. 2007;119(4):924–9.
5. Ibrahim SA, Kwoh CK, Krishnan E. Factors associated with patients who leave acute-care hospitals against medical advice. Am J Public Health 2007 Dec [cited 2017 Jan 5];97(12):2204–8. Available from: http://www.ncbi.nlm.nih.gov/pubmed/17971552.
6. Southern WN, Nahvi S, Arnsten JH. Increased risk of mortality and readmission among patients discharged against medical advice. Am J Med. 2012;125(6):594–602. Available from: https://doi.org/10.1016/j.amjmed.2011.12.017
7. Jerrard DA, Chasm RM. Patients leaving against medical advice (AMA) from the emergency department-disease prevalence and willingness to return. J Emerg Med. 2011;41(4):412–7. Available from: https://doi.org/10.1016/j.jemermed.2009.10.022
8. Franks P, Meldrum S, Fiscella K. Discharges against medical advice: are race/ethnicity predictors? J Gen Intern Med. 2006;21(9):955–60. Available from: https://doi.org/10.1007/BF02743144
9. Stearns CR, Bakamjian A, Sattar S, Weintraub MR. Discharges against medical advice at a county hospital: provider perceptions and practice. J Hosp Med. 2017;12(1):11–7. Available from: http://www.ncbi.nlm.nih.gov/pubmed/28125826
10. Kumar B, Deep KS. Discharge against medical advice: approaching a frustratingly common situation. 2015;113. Available from: http://www.kumarmd.org/wp-content/uploads/2015/07/Discharge-Against-Medical-Advice-Approaching-a-Frustratingly-Common-Situation.pdf.
11. Brofenbrenner U. Toward an experimental ecology of human development. Am Psychol. 1977;32(7):513–31.
12. Golden SD, Earp JA. Social ecological approaches to individuals and their contexts: twenty years of health education & behavior health promotion interventions. Health Educ Behav. 2012;39(3):364–72.
13. Weingart SN, Davis RB, Phillips RS. Patients discharged against medical advice from a general medicine service. J Gen Intern Med 1998 [cited 2017 Jan 5];13(8):568–71. Available from: http://www.pubmedcentral.nih.gov/articlerender.fcgi?artid=1496999&tool=pmcentrez&rendertype=abstract.
14. Spooner KK, Salemi JL, Salihu HM, Zoorob RJ. Discharge against medical advice in the United States, 2002–2011. Mayo Clin Proc. 2017;92(4):525–35. Available from: http://linkinghub.elsevier.com/retrieve/pii/S0025619617300733
15. Jeremiah J, O'Sullivan P, Stein MD. Who leaves against medical advice? J Gen Intern Med 1995 Jul [cited 2017 Jan 5];10(7):403–5. Available from: http://www.ncbi.nlm.nih.gov/pubmed/7472691.
16. Onukwugha E, Saunders E, Mullins CD, Pradel FG, Zuckerman M, Loh FE, et al. A qualitative study to identify reasons for discharges against medical advice in the cardiovascular setting. BMJ Open. 2012;2(4). Available from: http://bmjopen.bmj.com/content/2/4/e000902.abstract.
17. Onukwugha E, Saunders E, Mullins CD, Pradel FG, Zuckerman M, Weir MR. Reasons for discharges against medical advice: a qualitative study. Qual Saf Health Care. 2010;19(5):420–4. Available from: http://qualitysafety.bmj.com/content/19/5/420.abstract
18. Alfandre DJ. "I'm going home": discharges against medical advice. Mayo Clin Proc 2009 Mar [cited 2016 Nov 7];84(3):255–60. Available from: http://www.ncbi.nlm.nih.gov/pubmed/19252113.
19. Green P, Watts D, Poole S, Dhopesh V. Why patients sign out against medical advice (AMA): factors motivating patients to sign out AMA. Am J Drug Alcohol Abuse 2004 [cited 2017 May 23];30(2):489–93. Available from: http://www.tandfonline.com/doi/full/10.1081/ADA-120037390.
20. Onukwugha E, Shaya FT, Saunders E, Weir MR. Ethnic disparities, hospital quality, and discharges against medical advice among patients with cardiovascular disease. Ethn Dis.

2009;19(2):172–8. Available from: https://www.ethndis.org/edonline/index.php/ethndis/pages/view/priorarchives

21. Brook M, Hilty DM, Liu W, Hu R, Frye MA. Discharge against medical advice from inpatient psychiatric treatment: a literature review. Psychiatr Serv 2006 [cited 2016 Dec 5];57(8):1192–8. Available from: http://www.ncbi.nlm.nih.gov/pubmed/16870972.

22. Tawk R, Freels S, Mullner R. Associations of mental, and medical illnesses with against medical advice discharges: the National Hospital Discharge Survey, 1988–2006. Admin Pol Ment Health Ment Health Serv Res 2013 Mar 6 [cited 2016 Nov 7];40(2):124–32. Available from: http://link.springer.com/10.1007/s10488-011-0382-8.

23. Reinke DA, Walker M, Boslaugh S, Hodge D 3rd. Predictors of pediatric emergency patients discharged against medical advice. Clin Pediatr (Phila). 2009;48(3):263–70.

24. Macrohon BC, Alfandre D, Sclar D, Robison L, Anis A, Sun H, et al. Pediatrician's perspectives on discharge against medical advice (DAMA) among pediatric patients: a qualitative study. BMC Pediatr 2012 Dec 18 [cited 2016 Nov 7];12(1):75. Available from: http://bmcpediatr.biomedcentral.com/articles/10.1186/1471-2431-12-75.

25. Tucker Edmonds B, Ahlberg C, McPherson K, Srinivas S, Lorch S. Predictors and adverse pregnancy outcomes associated with antepartum discharge against medical advice. Matern Child Health J. 2014;18(3):640–7.

26. Fiscella K, Meldrum S, Franks P. Postpartum discharge against medical advice: who leaves and does it matter? Matern Child Health J. 2007;11(5):431–6.

27. Aliyu ZY. Discharge against medical advice: sociodemographic, clinical and financial perspectives. Int J Clin Pract 2002 Jun [cited 2017 May 23];56(5):325–7. Available from: http://www.ncbi.nlm.nih.gov/pubmed/12137437.

28. Grossman M. On the concept of health capital and the demand for health. J Political Econ 1972 Mar [cited 2017 May 20];80(2):223–55. Available from: http://www.journals.uchicago.edu/doi/10.1086/259880.

29. Ormel J, Lindenberg S, Steverink N, Vonkorff M. Quality of life and social production functions: a framework for understanding health effects. Soc Sci Med 1997 [cited 2017 May 20];45(7):1051–63. Available from: http://ac.els-cdn.com/S0277953697000324/1-s2.0-S0277953697000324-main.pdf?_tid=d8a3a904-3d96-11e7-9980-00000aab0f27&acdnat=1495310554_7627b547e25e0071a8c8c3f46ba992f0.

30. Pescosolido BA. Beyond rational choice: the social dynamics of how people seek help. Am J Sociol 1992 Jan [cited 2017 May 20];97(4):1096–138. Available from: http://www.journals.uchicago.edu/doi/10.1086/229863.

31. Windish DM, Ratanawongsa N. Providers' perceptions of relationships and professional roles when caring for patients who leave the hospital against medical advice. J Gen Intern Med. 2008;23(10):1698–707.

32. Yamagishi K. When a 12.86% mortality is more dangerous than 24.14%: implications for risk communication. Appl Cogn Psychol 1997 Dec [cited 2017 May 20];11(6):495–506. Available from: http://doi.wiley.com/10.1002/%28SICI%291099-0720%28199712%2911%3A6%3C495%3A%3AAID-ACP481%3E3.0.CO%3B2-J.

33. Hendrickx L, Vlek C, Oppewal H. Relative importance of scenario information and frequency information in the judgment of risk. Acta Psychol 1989 [cited 2017 May 20];72(1):41–63. Available from: http://www.sciencedirect.com/science/article/pii/0001691889900504.

34. Hibbard JH, Peters E. Supporting informed consumer health care decisions: data presentation approaches that facilitate the use of information in choice. Annu Rev Public Health 2003 Jan [cited 2017 May 20];24(1):413–33. Available from: http://www.annualreviews.org/doi/10.1146/annurev.publhealth.24.100901.141005.

35. Kaplan RM, Hammel B, Sehimmel LE. Patient information processing and the decision to accept treatment. [cited 2017 May 20]; Available from: http://rmkaplan.bol.ucla.edu/Robert_M._Kaplan/1985_Publications_files/0093.pdf.

36. Jahangir E, Irazola V, Rubinstein A, Wright J, Williams R, Wilkinson J, et al. Need, enabling, predisposing, and behavioral determinants of access to preventative care in Argentina: analysis of the National Survey of Risk Factors. In: Barengo NC, editor. PLoS One [cited 2017 Jan 7];7(9):e45053. Available from: http://dx.plos.org/10.1371/journal.pone.0045053.

37. Blanchard J, Nayar S, Lurie N. Patient-provider and patient-staff racial concordance and perceptions of mistreatment in the health care setting. J Gen Intern Med 2007 Jul 5 [cited 2017 Jan 5];22(8):1184–9. Available from: http://www.ncbi.nlm.nih.gov/pubmed/17486386.
38. Blanchard J, Lurie N. R-E-S-P-E-C-T: patient reports of disrespect in the health care setting and its impact on care. J Fam Pract 2004 Sep [cited 2017 Jan 5];53(9):721–30. Available from: http://www.ncbi.nlm.nih.gov/pubmed/15353162.
39. Saitz R. Discharges against medical advice: time to address the causes. CMAJ. 2002;167(6): 647–8.
40. Alfandre D. Reconsidering against medical advice discharges: embracing patient-centeredness to promote high quality care and a renewed research agenda. J Gen Intern Med. 2013;28(12):1657–62.
41. Clark MA, Abbott JT, Adyanthaya T. Ethics seminars: a best-practice approach to navigating the against-medical-advice discharge. Acad Emerg Med. 2014;21(9):1050–7.
42. Devitt PJ, Devitt AC, Dewan M. Does identifying a discharge as "Against Medical Advice" confer legal protection? J Fam Pract. 2000;49(3):224–7.
43. Schaefer GR, Matus H, Schumann JH, Sauter K, Vekhter B, Meltzer DO, et al. Financial responsibility of hospitalized patients who left against medical advice: medical urban legend? J Gen Intern Med. 2012;27(7):825–30.
44. Feng Z, Wright B, Mor V. Sharp rise in Medicare enrollees being held in hospitals for observation raises concerns about causes and consequences. Health Aff (Millwood) 2012 Jun 1 [cited 2017 Aug 10];31(6):1251–9. Available from: http://www.ncbi.nlm.nih.gov/pubmed/22665837.
45. Public Policy Committee. The observation status problem. J Hosp Med. 2012;7(S2):1–1. Available from: http://doi.wiley.com/10.1002/jhm.1927
46. Sheehy AM, Graf B, Gangireddy S, Hoffman R, Ehlenbach M, Heidke C, et al. Hospitalized but not admitted: characteristics of patients with "observation status" at an academic medical center. JAMA Intern Med 2013 Nov 25 [cited 2017 Jun 1];173(21):1991–8. Available from: http://www.ncbi.nlm.nih.gov/pubmed/23835927.
47. Horwitz L, Partovian C, Lin Z, Herrin J, Grady J, Conover M, et al. Hospital-wide (all-condition) 30-day risk-standardized readmission measure DRAFT measure methodology report submitted by Yale New Haven Health Services Corporation/Center for Outcomes Research & Evaluation (YNHHSC/CORE). [cited 2017 Apr 3]; Available from: https://www.cms.gov/Medicare/Quality-Initiatives-Patient-Assessment-Instruments/MMS/downloads/MMSHospital-WideAll-ConditionReadmissionRate.pdf.
48. Horwitz LI, Partovian C, Lin Z, Grady JN, Herrin J, Conover M, et al. Development and use of an administrative claims measure for profiling hospital-wide performance on 30-day unplanned readmission. Ann Intern Med 2014 Nov 18 [cited 2017 Apr 3];161(10_Supplement):S66–75. Available from: http://www.ncbi.nlm.nih.gov/pubmed/25402406.
49. CMS. Medicare enrollment charts – chronic conditions data warehouse [Internet]. Available from: https://www.ccwdata.org/web/guest/medicare-charts/medicare-enrollment-charts.
50. CMS. Medicaid enrollment charts – chronic conditions data warehouse [Internet]. [cited 2017 Jun 1]. Available from: https://www.ccwdata.org/web/guest/medicaid-charts.
51. van Walraven C, Jennings A, Forster AJ. A meta-analysis of hospital 30-day avoidable readmission rates. J Eval Clin Pract. 2012;18(6):1211–8.
52. Vest JR, Gamm LD, Oxford BA, Gonzalez MI, Slawson KM, Jencks S, et al. Determinants of preventable readmissions in the United States: a systematic review. Implement Sci. 2010; 5(1):88. Available from: http://implementationscience.biomedcentral.com/articles/10.1186/1748-5908-5-88
53. Thompson MP, Waters TM, Kaplan CM, Cao Y, Bazzoli GJ. Most hospitals received annual penalties for excess readmissions, but some fared better than others. Health Aff (Millwood). 2017;36(5):893–901. Available from: http://content.healthaffairs.org/lookup/doi/10.1377/hlthaff.2016.1204
54. Gu Q, Koenig L, Faerberg J, Steinberg CR, Vaz C, Wheatley MP. The medicare hospital readmissions reduction program: potential unintended consequences for hospitals serving vulnerable populations. Health Serv Res. 2014;49(3):818–37.

55. Lorenz TH, Green JM, Lewis WC, Stone M, Calden G, Thurston JR. Investigation of irregular discharge of tuberculous patients; a special ward procedure for reducing against-medical-advice discharges. Am Rev Tuber U S. 1955;72(5):633–46.
56. Zumla A, Nahid P, Cole ST. Advances in the development of new tuberculosis drugs and treatment regimens. Nat Rev Drug Discov 2013 Apr 30 [cited 2017 May 23];12(5):388–404. Available from: http://www.nature.com/doifinder/10.1038/nrd4001.
57. Brush RW, Kaelbling R. Discharge of psychiatric patients against medical advice. J Nerv Ment Dis U S. 1963;136:288–92.
58. Levine J, Monroe JJ. Discharge of narcotic drug addicts against medical advice. Public Health Rep. 1964;79:13–8.
59. Lewis JM. Discharge against medical advice. The doctor's role. Hosp Community Psychiatry. 1966;17(9):266–70.
60. Miles JE, Adlersberg M, Reith G, Cumming J. Discharges against medical advice from voluntary psychiatric units. Hosp Community Psychiatry. 1976;27(12):859–64.
61. Jankowski CB, Drum DE. Diagnostic correlates of discharge against medical advice. Arch Gen Psychiatry. 1977;34(2):153–5. Available from: http://www.ncbi.nlm.nih.gov/pubmed/843174
62. Smith DB, Telles JL. Discharges against medical advice at regional acute care hospitals. Am J Public Health 1991 Feb [cited 2017 Jan 25];81(2):212–15. Available from: http://ajph.apha-publications.org/doi/10.2105/AJPH.81.2.212.
63. Moy E, Bartman BA. Race and hospital discharge against medical advice. J Natl Med Assoc. 1996;88(10):658–60.

Chapter 3
Legal Considerations of Patient Refusals of Treatment Against Medical Advice

Arthur R. Derse

Informed Consent and Refusal

In most circumstances of medical treatment, before treatment of a patient may be begun, the patient must give permission for treatment [1]. This requirement is supported by the ethical principle of autonomy in which an individual should have the choice whether to accept a proposed treatment, even if the treatment appears to be in the patient's best interests [2]. This requirement is also mediated by the legal principle of the necessity of consent for patient treatment, first stated over a century ago that "[e]very human being of adult years and sound mind has a right to determine what shall be done with his own body…" and violations may be liable for damages [3]. This legal principle of required consent for patient treatment was further extended over a half-century ago to include "material" information that must be disclosed to the patient in order to make the decision. The material information must include risks and benefits, alternatives, and the consequences of choosing to forgo treatment [4]. Depending upon the jurisdiction, the standard for what information must be disclosed is either what the average prudent physician would disclose to the patient (the professional standard) [5] or what information the objective patient would find material to make the decision (the reasonable patient standard) [6].

Consent may be waived by the patient through words (e.g., "Do whatever you think is best, doctor"), with the proviso that the patient should be informed that he or she has the right to be informed of the risks, benefits, alternatives, and choice of no treatment. The patient should also be informed that he or she may resume decision-making when wished. Consent may also be implied by the patient if the patient's actions make such an inference reasonable [7].

A. R. Derse (✉)
Center for Bioethics and Medical Humanities, Institute for Health and Equity, and
Department of Emergency Medicine, Medical College of Wisconsin, Milwaukee, WI, USA
e-mail: aderse@mcw.edu

© Springer International Publishing AG, part of Springer Nature 2018
D. Alfandre (ed.), *Against-Medical-Advice Discharges from the Hospital*,
https://doi.org/10.1007/978-3-319-75130-6_3

Consent may also be forgone during an emergency. This legal exception is known as the "emergency privilege," specific to life- or limb-threatening emergencies. Along with the emergent condition, the other requirements for the exception include the lack of a legally authorized decision-maker and the likelihood (if known) that this individual would consent or a reasonable person would consent ("presumed consent") [8].

Some emergencies will fulfill each of the requirements of the emergency exception for informed consent. In those circumstances, consent by the patient may be forgone. An example would be a patient who arrives to the emergency department unresponsive without a legally authorized decision-maker readily available. However, even if a medical situation is emergent, if the patient has the capacity to make a medical decision, or if a legal representative is readily available to make the decision, then the emergency exception to informed consent would not apply. For many non-emergent cases of patient refusal of treatment, the need for medical treatment does not supersede the right of a patient with the capacity to make a decision to exercise that right of consent or refusal.

If the patient has the capacity to refuse or consent to medical treatment, this requirement for consent applies even when the treatment would save the life of the patient. Patients have won the legal right to refuse life-sustaining medical treatment, whether this be in the form of cardiopulmonary resuscitation, ventilation, blood transfusions, or nutrition and hydration. This right is grounded in the liberty interest of the due process clause of the Fourteenth Amendment of the US Constitution [9]. The mere fact that the patient may die because of the refusal is not enough to be able to force the patient to accept treatment [10]. A classic case is that of the adult Jehovah's Witness patient who refuses a lifesaving blood transfusion. Although a half-century ago, courts supported an intervention on the part of physicians who wished to administer a blood transfusion, reasoning that physicians had a duty to prevent the individual from suicidal actions [11], more recent court decisions have supported the right of the patient who possesses decision-making capacity to refuse life-sustaining medical treatment in the form of transfusions [12, 13].

Decision-Making Capacity: The Central Question in Patient Refusal

Decision-making capacity is the ability of the individual to make decisions about medical care. Decision-making capacity should be differentiated from legal competence: a person is presumed to be legally competent until proven otherwise, and if found incompetent by a court, a guardian (or in some jurisdictions, a conservator) will be appointed to make personal decisions, financial decisions, or both. Decision-making capacity is specific to the medical choice to be made and depends upon the individual abilities of the patient, the requirements of the task, and the consequences of the decision [14]. When the consequences are substantial, there is greater need for certainty of the ability of the patient to make the decision.

Decision-making capacity consists of three major components: (1) the ability to understand the information about the medical situation and to understand and appreciate the consequences of the choice to be made, (2) the ability to evaluate the choices comparing risks and benefits of the choices and to make a rational choice (supported by consistency over time), and (3) the ability to communicate that choice to the treatment team [15].

Though patients with decision-making capacity have secured the legal right to refuse potentially life-sustaining treatment, a patient's refusal does not end the professional and legal obligations of the physician. When a patient who can make decisions about medical treatment refuses a recommended medical intervention, the physician has the legal duty to inform the patient of the consequences of that refusal, i.e., to allow the patient to make what is known as an "informed refusal." The principle of informed refusal is a correlative obligation to that of informed consent. A patient's right to information about a proposed treatment includes a patient's right to learn the consequences of the alternative of forgoing treatment. The patient may also waive the right to be informed of the consequences [16].

Some observers have criticized physicians for paternalism in questioning a patient's decision-making capacity when a patient refuses a recommended treatment, but not questioning the patient's decision-making capacity if the patient agrees with that recommendation [17]. However, a more benign interpretation of this paradox is that physicians generally recommend treatments that are in the best interests of patients or in accord with the patient's long-standing wishes. When the stakes are high, in that the treatment proposed may be the standard of care and refusal may have life-threatening implications, it may be argued that the physician has a correspondingly heightened duty to assure that the patient has the capacity to refuse and to understand the implications of the refusal [18]. If a person with decision-making capacity has the right to refuse life-sustaining medical treatment, when a patient refuses that life-sustaining medical treatment, the determination of decision-making capacity becomes a crucial element in making sure that the patient's choice is an autonomous one. This responsibility is weighty for emergency physicians, intensivists, or surgeons who do not have a long-standing relationship with the patient in which the values of the patient are well known and the refusal can be understood within those values.

Assessment of patient decision-making capacity at a basic level is a skill required of all clinicians, since possession of decision-making capacity is a fundamental requirement for informed consent and refusal by the patient of proposed interventions and treatment. However, in complex or difficult cases when decision-making capacity is at issue, mental health professionals, including psychiatrists and neuropsychologists, may be of value in helping to make this determination. However, in the emergency situation, a specialist consultation may not be available, and the physician may need to make this evaluation.

There are widely used tests for determining decision-making capacity that include the Mini-Mental Status Exam (MMSE) [19] and the Montreal Cognitive

Assessment (MoCA) [20], which can give an overall score that may aid in determining decision-making capacity (especially if there are very low scores), though there is no recognized "gold standard" test for decision-making capacity [21]. It should be noted that a lack of decision-making capacity may be temporary, and it may be that patients need more information to be able to make a decision [22]. Even with cognitive impairment, some patients may still be able to make a decision about basic medical decisions. A psychiatric diagnosis does not preclude the possession of decision-making capacity [23].

Thus, the central issue in patient refusal may hinge not on whether the patient has the legal right to refuse but whether or not the patient has decision-making capacity to exercise that right. If the patient does have decision-making capacity, the patient can refuse life-sustaining medical treatment with the proviso that the patient should have an opportunity to understand the risks and consequences of refusal of treatment. If the patient does not have decision-making capacity, then the patient does not have the ability to exercise the right to make an informed refusal.

When the patient does not have this decision-making capacity, if this is an emergency (in that there is a life or limb threat) and time is of the essence and a reasonable person would consent, then the emergency exception to informed consent would apply, and the physician should act in the best interests of the patient and concurrently seek a decision-maker. If this is not an emergency, and the patient is under the legal protection of guardianship or has a health-care agent designated by a power of attorney for health care, a discussion with the guardian or agent should be undertaken.

If the patient does not have decision-making capacity, for instance because of either a psychiatric disease or impairment from intoxicants, the patient cannot make a valid refusal (or, for that matter, acceptance) of medical treatment. Treatment may be administered under the emergency exception to informed consent.

Where the medical situation is not emergent, but there may be a risk to self or others, pertinent emergency detention and treatment statutes may be invoked. An example of such a case is when an emergency physician encounters a patient who came to the emergency department by automobile and is intoxicated to such an extent that he or she has lost the ability to make medical decisions, with no one available to supervise the patient or make sure the patient does not drive a motor vehicle. The medical situation is not emergent, but there is the potential of danger. In many cases the prudent course might be to detain the patient temporarily until he or she regains decision-making capacity and the ability to drive without impairment. In a nonemergency situation without an imminent danger of harm to self or others, refusal of treatment should be respected, though mental health attention or an engagement of adult protective services may be warranted. Where the patient has a guardian or a health-care agent from a power of attorney document that has been activated, treatment options should be presented to the legal health-care decision-maker.

Refusal to Allow the Physician to Determine Decision-Making Capacity

If the patient who refuses emergent or urgently needed treatment also refuses to allow the physician to make an assessment of whether the patient can make such a decision, the physician is faced with the dilemma of whether to accept that refusal. Unless there are indications otherwise, under most circumstances, patients may be presumed to have decision-making capacity until an examination that includes an evaluation of decision-making capacity confirms or contradicts this. Since decision-making capacity is essential, the physician should make the best attempt to engage with the patient and persuade the patient to allow that examination. Often engagement and persuasion may work.

When engagement and persuasion do not work, can the physician temporarily detain and even restrain the patient to make a determination of decision-making capacity? Restraining a patient temporarily to determine whether the patient has the decision-making capacity to refuse treatment may seem like an oxymoron. However, if the physician is unsure of the patient's capacity to make a medical decision, the physician may have to weigh which course of action is better: to detain the patient with the least forceful means for a short period as possible in which decision-making capacity can be determined or to take the risk that the patient be allowed to leave when evidence of the patient's ability to be able to make this decision was not ascertained. If the patient subsequently dies or has a serious outcome, the latter course may be the more difficult to justify. Survivors, or those who have been subsequently injured by a patient who was allowed to leave, may argue that the patient did not have the capacity to make the decision, so should have been restrained as a danger to himself or herself and treated despite refusal [24]. Many of these kinds of cases are litigated in trial courts but are not published in appellate reports, so not widely known [25]. The physician should consider in advance this dilemma and consult with legal counsel about better ethical and legal approaches in the jurisdiction.

However, if the patient is not determined to pose an imminent threat to oneself or others, in at least one state, the patient may have the right to leave without detention or treatment, even if an injury to the patient later occurs. In Kowalski v. St. Francis Hospital and Health Centers [26], the New York Court of Appeals held in a divided opinion that a patient with severe intoxication (blood alcohol level of 0.369%) had the right to leave against medical advice without a corresponding duty on the part of the emergency physician to detain him. The patient, who was not determined by the emergency physician to be a danger to self or others, had originally agreed to go to a detoxification center, but left the waiting area, and within hours was hit by a car and severely injured. The patient made a claim of a failed duty by the emergency physician to detain him on the basis of potential harm to self. The court found that the emergency physician did not have such a duty in the circumstances of the case. Physicians may interpret this case as giving wide latitude for patients to refuse treatment. However, there are several caveats about this case. First, this New York case is not controlling in other states where the duty of care might be found to have more broadly required protection of the patient or others from potential harm. Second, in this case, the patient presented to the emergency department voluntarily, not through law enforcement escort as a potential danger to self. Third, the emergency physician did not determine that the patient was a danger to self or others and, assuming that determination was accurate at the time, had no duty to detain the patient involuntarily. The same case may well have come out the opposite way in a different state's jurisdiction.

Documentation of Patient Refusal and Understanding

The issues of documentation of refusal and its legal implications arise in these cases. Many of these so-called "against medical advice (AMA)" forms document the patient's refusal of hospitalization or treatment and include spaces to fill in information disclosed of risks and consequences, as well as places for signatures of patients and, in some cases, witnesses to the discussion. Some of these forms also state that the patient hereby waives his or her right to sue for damages for potential injuries that he or she may suffer as a consequence of the refusal of medical treatment. Depending upon state law, this broad waiver of legal rights may not be valid [27]. However, even though a signed AMA form by itself may not be legally protective for the physician or institution, it may serve as evidence that an attempt was made to persuade the patient to accept treatment and that the patient was informed of the risks of refusal with support by a witness who can attest to this conversation [28].

Whether there is an AMA form signed by the patient or not, there should be documentation in the patient's chart of the patient's refusal, as well as the evaluation by the physician that the patient had the decision-making capacity to refuse treatment. The form itself will not be helpful if the patient who signed the form lacked the decision-making capacity to refuse and, if not waived by the patient, to be provided the information necessary to make an informed refusal [29]. The physician should also make sure the patient knows (and should document) that the patient may return at any time for treatment.

There is a danger of reliance on the completion of the form as the fulfillment of the obligation of obtaining an informed refusal. Just as an informed consent form should not replace the required conversation between doctor and patient about medical treatment, so also an AMA form should not replace the required offer – and provision if allowed – of information of the consequences of refusal. Additionally, it should be noted that the production of such a form may further impede communication with the patient by raising distrust of the physician's motives for the documentation.

Some administrative bodies may require patient (or surrogate) signature of refusal of treatment or, in its absence, specific documentation of the patient or representative's declination to sign the form acknowledging the refusal of treatment. For instance, hospitals have responsibilities under the Emergency Medical Treatment and Labor Act (EMTALA) [30] to evaluate patients who present to the emergency department with a medical screening examination to determine whether they have an emergency medical condition (EMC) and to treat the patients, or stabilize and transfer them appropriately to another institution that can provide the needed emergency treatment. The Centers for Medicare and Medicaid Services (CMS) issued interpretive guidelines concerning responsibilities of Medicare-participating hospitals in emergency cases that state:

> In cases where an individual (or person acting in the individual's behalf) withdrew the initial request for a medical screening examination (MSE) and/or treatment for an EMC and demanded his or her transfer, or demanded to leave the hospital, look for a signed informed refusal of examination and treatment form by either the individual or a person acting on the individual's behalf. ... If the individual (or person acting in the individual's behalf) refused to sign the consent form, look for documentation by the hospital personnel that states that the individual refused to sign the form. The fact that an individual has not signed the form is not, however, automatically a violation of the screening requirement. Hospitals must, under the regulations, use their best efforts to obtain a signature from an individual refusing further care. [31]

In light of these kinds of regulatory guidelines, a signature may be sought as a documented acknowledgment of a patient's voluntary and informed refusal. In lieu of that signature, there should be documentation of the elements of refusal and information by the health-care providers.

Physicians have sometimes asserted that a patient who refuses a complete treatment course (e.g., hospitalization and treatment with IV antibiotics) should not be offered partial treatment (e.g., oral antibiotics only), since if partial treatment is not the standard of care, it might result in liability for substandard care. However, if partial treatment might be of benefit to the patient, the record of that treatment may be allowed as evidence of the physician's willingness to provide at least a level of treatment, even if substandard, that the patient was willing to accept [32].

Adolescents: Mature and Emancipated Minors

As a general rule, except in an emergency, informed consent for treatment of a minor must be obtained from the parent or guardian of the minor. However, if a parent or guardian refuses treatment, federal and state law may override a parent's refusal of treatment when that treatment is clearly in the best interests of the child. In an emergency, treatment of children in their best interests when there is no parent or guardian is warranted under the emergency privilege to informed consent. The law recognizes that under certain medical conditions, an adolescent minor may make a medical decision independent of parent or guardian. Consent by adolescents is generally allowed for treatments such as for STIs, HIV, and AIDS, contraception, mental health, and alcohol and drug abuse [33].

Emancipation is the state of legal independence of the minor from parents or guardian to make decisions in the same way an adult may do so. Emancipation is presumed at the age of majority set by the state but may be determined earlier by statute or common law. Approximately half of states designate emancipation by statute and others by common law in response to a petition of emancipation. Common emancipation landmarks include marriage, military enlistment, self-support or living apart from parents, completion of a secondary education, and, in some states, giving birth to, or fathering, a child. A court may grant emancipation for a specific purpose such as refusal of medical treatment [34].

A mature minor is defined as a minor who, though not emancipated, is determined to be able to accept or refuse proposed health intervention or treatment (with or without the knowledge or consent of parents). Mature minor status may be determined by a court, a statute, or regulation. Mature minor status may be used to protect the confidentiality of a doctor-adolescent patient relationship or may also be used as a defense by a health-care provider from criminal or civil battery or other claims arising from a mature minor's consent for that intervention [35]. However, for medical decisions in most jurisdictions, even if the minor is considered cognitively mature, unless the minor has been adjudicated as mature as a matter of law, parental consent is still required [36].

Emancipated minors may refuse medical treatment under the same circumstances in which an adult may do so. Mature minors may be found by courts to be able to refuse life-sustaining medical treatment, especially if there is parental support for the refusal. For instance, in Virginia, a 16-year-old boy with Hodgkin's lymphoma who had been treated with one round of chemotherapy had a remission and recurrence. The adolescent patient with parental concurrence refused a second treatment even though the treatment was highly likely to be effective in treating this life-threatening condition. Although the state charged the parents with neglect and attempted to remove him from their custody, the court sided with the adolescent and parents in support of the refusal. Virginia subsequently passed a statute that allows teenagers 14 years old or older who are sufficiently mature (and with good faith concurrence of their parents or guardians) to refuse medical treatments. They may seek alternative treatments so long as they have considered all other medical options [37].

However, in a similar case, the Connecticut Supreme Court in 2015 affirmed that a 17-year-old girl with Hodgkin's lymphoma who had been treated with two rounds of chemotherapy but with her mother's concurrence had refused subsequent treatment was deemed by a trial court not to be a mature minor capable of refusing treatment. Note that in both these cases, the likelihood of the 5-year survival with treatment was between 85% and 90%. Death was highly likely without the treatment. The Connecticut Supreme Court affirmed the forced treatment with chemotherapy over the objections of both the patient and the mother. These contrasting cases show that depending upon the jurisdiction, medical intervention that is seen to be in the best interests of the adolescent with a high degree of likelihood of success may be judged differently by courts as to whether or not these adolescents are mature minors that may refuse medical treatment [38].

Thus, though adolescents generally have established legal rights to accept some beneficial medical treatment independent of parents or guardians, depending upon state law, parental consent may still be required, and even with parental support of the refusal, adolescents may not have a corresponding right to refuse that beneficial treatment.

Summary

Patients who refuse medical treatment that appears to be both necessary and in their best interests pose a vexing medical, ethical, and legal challenge. US law recognizes the right of the person to refuse treatment, including life-sustaining medical treatment based in the liberty interest of the due process clause of the Fourteenth Amendment of the US Constitution. However, when the stakes are high, the central question is whether the individual has the required capacity to be able to exercise his or her right to make the pertinent medical decision. When there is a question about the patient's required decision-making capacity, an assessment of the capacity should be made and documented. A written form that documents the patient's refusal of treatment against medical advice (AMA form) may not necessarily be legally protective in itself but may be useful as evidence of the patient's refusal, understanding, and voluntariness with documentation of witnesses to the discussion. Although adults have the right to refuse life-sustaining medical treatment, federal and state laws may override parents' refusal of treatment for their children. Depending upon state law, some adolescents have rights to make their own decisions to accept certain beneficial treatments; however, their right to refuse life-sustaining medical treatment may be circumscribed.

References

1. Derse AR, Schiedermayer D. Practical ethics for students, interns, and residents. 4th. Hagerstown, Maryland: University Publishing Group; 2015. Ch III, Informed Consent, p. 18–20.
2. Beauchamp TL, Childress JF. Respect for autonomy, Ch. 4. In: Principles of biomedical ethics. 7th ed. New York: Oxford University Press; 2013. p. 101–49.
3. Schloendorff v. Society of New York Hospital, 105 N.E. 92 (N.Y. 1914) at 93, 211 N.Y. 125.
4. Salgo v. Leland Stanford Jr. Board of Trustees, 154 Cal.App.2d 560, 317 P.2d 170. 1957.
5. Natanson v. Kline 186 Kan. 393, 350 P.2d 1093. 1960.
6. Canterbury v. Spence. 464 F.2d 772, U.S. Ct. App. D.C. Cir. (D.C. Cir. 1972).
7. O'Brien v. Cunard S.S. Co. 154 Mass. 272, 28 N.E. 266. Mass. 1891.
8. Prosser and Keeton on Torts. 5th ed. Consent: emergency privilege. 1984, p. 117–8.
9. Cruzan v. Director of Missouri department of Health. 497 U.S. 261, 110 S.Ct. 2841, 111 L.Ed. 2d. 224. 1990.
10. Meisel A. Legal myths about terminating life support. Arch Intern Med. 1991;151:1497–502.
11. Application of the President and Directors of Georgetown College, Inc. 331 F.2d 1000 (D.C. Cir. 1964).
12. Fosmire v. Nicoleau. 551 N.E.2d 77, 80 (N.Y. 1990).
13. Wons v. Public Health Trust of Dade County. 500 So.2d 679 (Fla.App. 3 Dist. 1987).
14. President's Commission for the Study of Ethical Problems in Medicine and Biomedical and Behavioral Research. Making health care decisions, vol. 1. Washington, DC: US Government Printing Office; 1992. p. 55–68.
15. Derse AR, Schiedermayer D. Practical ethics for students, interns, and residents. 4th ed. Hagerstown, Maryland: University Publishing Group. 2015. Ch. IV, Competence and decision-making capacity. p. 21–24.
16. Truman v. Thomas. 27 Cal.3d, 285, 165 Cal.Rptr. 308, 611 P.2d 902. 1980.

17. Roth LH, Meisel A, Lidz CW. Tests of competency to consent to treatment. Am J Psychiatry. 1977;134:279–84.
18. Derse AR. What part of "no" don't you understand? Patient refusal of recommended treatment in the emergency department. Mt Sinai J Med. 2005;72(4):221–7.
19. Folstein MF, Folstein SE, McHugh PR. "Mini-mental state." A practical method for grading the cognitive state of patients for the clinician. J Psychiatr Res. 1975;12(3):189–98.
20. Nasreddine ZS, Phillips NA, Bedirian V, Charbonneau S, Whitehead V, Collin I, et al. The Montreal cognitive assessment, MoCA: a brief screening tool for mild cognitive impairment. J Am Geriatr Soc. 2005;53(4):695–9.
21. Appelbaum PS. Assessment of patient's competence to consent to treatment. N Engl J Med. 2007;357:1834–40.
22. Ganzini L, Volicer L, Nelson WA, Fox E, Derse AR. Ten myths about decision-making capacity. J Am Med Dir Assoc. 2005;6:S100–4.
23. Ganzini L, Volicer L, Nelson WA, Derse AR. Pitfalls in assessment of decision-making capacity. Psychosomatics. 2003;44:237–43.
24. Raines RT. Evaluating the inebriated: an analysis of the HIPAA privacy rule and its implications for intoxicated patients in emergency departments. Univ Dayton Law Rev. 2016;40(3):479–98.
25. Does ED chart leave AMA patient free to claim. 'If Only I'd Known the Risks?' ED Leg Lett. 2017;29(2):20–2.
26. Kowalski v. St. Francis Hospital and Health Centers, 2013 N.Y. LEXIS 1677 (N.Y. Ct. App. June 26, 2013), 2013 WL 3197637, 2013 N.Y. Slip Op. 05437 (2d Dept. July 24, 2013).
27. Patient's signature on AMA form won't stop successful lawsuit. Emergency department legal letter. AHC Media. 2016:129–131.
28. Levy F, Mareiniss DP, Iacovelli C. The importance of a proper against-medical-advice (AMA) discharge: how signing out AMA may create significant liability protection for providers. Am J Emerg Med. 2012;43(3):516–20.
29. Alfandre D, Schumann J. What is wrong with discharges against medical advice (and how to fix them). JAMA. 2013;310(22):2393–4.
30. Examination and treatment for emergency medical conditions and women in labor. 42 U.S. Code § 1395dd.
31. Centers for Medicare and Medicaid Services. Emergency Medical Treatment & Labor Act (EMTALA). State operations manual appendix V – interpretive guidelines – responsibilities of Medicare participating hospitals in emergency cases. (Rev. 60, 07–16-10). https://www.cms.gov/Regulations-and-Guidance/Legislation/EMTALA.
32. Marco CM, Brenner JM, Kraus C, McGrath N, Derse AR. Refusal of emergency medical treatment: case studies and ethical foundations. Ann Emerg Med. 2017;70:696–703.
33. National Association of District Attorneys. Minor consent to medical treatment laws. 2013. http://www.ndaa.org/pdf/Minor%20Consent%20to%20Medical%20Treatment%20(2).pdf.
34. Michon K. Emancipation of minors. NOLO Press. http://www.nolo.com/legal-encyclopedia/emancipation-of-minors-32237.html.
35. Schlam L, Wood JP. Informed consent to the medical treatment of minors: law & practice. 10 Health Matrix 2000; 141 Available at: http://scholarlycommons.law.case.edu/healthmatrix/vol10/iss2/3.
36. Coleman DL, Rosoff PM. The legal authority of mature minors to consent to general medical treatment. Pediatrics. 2013;131(4):786–93.
37. CHAPTER 597 An Act to amend and reenact § 63.2-100 of the Code of Virginia, relating to abused or neglected children. [S 905] Approved March 20, 2007.
38. In re: Cassandra C. (SC 19426) Conn. 2015.

Chapter 4
Ethical Considerations in Against Medical Advice Discharges: Value Conflicts Over Patient Autonomy and Best Interests

Jeffrey T. Berger and David Alfandre

AMA discharges occur when a physician formally recognizes and documents a capacitated patient's choice to both decline further inpatient medical care and leave the hospital prior to a recommended clinical endpoint. The phrase "discharge against medical advice" (AMA) is well established in the clinical vernacular, and these irregular discharges have been described in the medical literature for at least 70 years. However, discharge AMA has been little considered from a bioethical perspective even though it is ethically complex. Moreover, confronting AMA discharges without an adequate understanding of the ethics can leave the clinician without a strong conceptual grounding for clinical management. In this chapter, we will review the central value conflict and evaluate the language used to describe this hospital-based phenomenon. We will also unpack various conceptual and factual assumptions embedded in AMA discharges and propose practical management strategies by examining some of the ethical principles that underlie the AMA problem.

Patients who wish to leave the hospital prior to a clinically specified endpoint present physicians with a common but challenging ethical dilemma. Physicians, as part of the legal and ethical informed consent process, are obligated to follow capacitated patient's wishes for the type of care they wish to receive. This obligation, which respects patient's autonomy, stems from patient's right to self-determination and their right to accept recommended care, as well as to decline it. Patients are

The views expressed in this article are those of the authors and do not necessarily reflect the position or policy of the U.S. Department of Veterans Affairs, the US Government, or the VA National Center for Ethics in Health Care.

J. T. Berger (✉)
Division of Palliative Medicine and Bioethics, Department of Medicine,
NYU Winthrop Hospital, Mineola, NY, USA
e-mail: jberger@winthrop.org

D. Alfandre
VHA National Center for Ethics in Health Care, Department of Veterans Affairs,
NYU School of Medicine, New York, NY, USA

© Springer International Publishing AG, part of Springer Nature 2018   41
D. Alfandre (ed.), *Against-Medical-Advice Discharges from the Hospital*,
https://doi.org/10.1007/978-3-319-75130-6_4

entitled to decide which care they wish to accept consistent with their values, needs, and preferences, whether that treatment is provided in the inpatient or outpatient setting, or whether it is a minor procedure or life-sustaining treatment.

Physicians also have a reciprocal fiduciary obligation to promote the patient's best interest by recommending medically appropriate care. When patients choose to decline recommended care, physicians may experience this refusal as their failure to provide beneficial, high-quality care. Thus, physicians may find themselves troubled by balancing these dual obligations of respecting patient's autonomy while simultaneously trying to promote their best interests. The most expedient way in which physicians resolve this ethical tension is to accept the primacy of the patient's right to autonomy, designate the discharge as AMA, and relinquish responsibility for a decision that may result in worse health and health service outcomes. However, there are numerous other more productive ways to resolve some of the ethical tension that results from trying to address conflicting ethical obligations. How best to honor these dual obligations is covered later in the chapter.

There are a number of factual and conceptual assumptions embedded in the descriptor "discharge AMA." The word choice of "discharge AMA" implies that (1) a physician has advised a specific medical plan for the patient and (2) the patient, at his or her behest, intends to leave the hospital having rejected this advice. Because the clinical and ethical realities of these situations are multifaceted, further examination of this language and assumptions can illuminate some broader perspectives that can lead to new solutions for this problem.

First is the use of institution- or physician-centric language with AMA discharges. Both colloquially and within the literature, patients are frequently described as "refusing care" or "threatening" to leave AMA or making "bad choices." This word choice communicates that the patient is inherently difficult and unworthy of consideration because they have articulated preferences inconsistent with the physician's recommendations. This pejorative word choice also may help to perpetuate the stigma of AMA discharges by framing the patient as unreasonable. This wording doesn't support a broader conception of a collaborative, inclusive process but rather suggests that the physician has all the information and power to make the final decision. Although more value-neutral language might include "patient-initiated discharge," that wording also falls short in that it neglects the critical role of professional judgment about medical suitability for discharge. Both patient and physician bring critical information to the discharge planning process. How that process is discussed and described in the medical record has consequences.

Unpacking the AMA discharge language leads us to consider a number of factual assumptions when there is a disagreement about discharge. They are as follows:

1. The patient has notified a member of the inpatient hospital staff that she/he wishes to leave the hospital.
2. In recognizing that the patient wishes to deviate from the originally agreed upon inpatient treatment plan, the physician develops and communicates a primary recommendation for continued hospitalization that is medically appropriate and reasonable.

3. Using information from the patient about their wish to leave the hospital, the physician makes efforts to develop and communicate medically sound and reasonable alternatives to the preferred primary recommendation, all of which include continued hospitalization.
4. The patient is capable of understanding, deliberating upon, and acting upon the recommendation(s).
5. The patient chooses to decline the physician's recommendations to remain hospitalized, and further negotiation does not alter the patient's original decision.
6. The physician accedes to the patient's request and formalizes the discharge as AMA by documenting the details of the declination of inpatient care in the patient's health record.

Apart from these factual assumptions are a number of conceptual assumptions implied in the language of "discharge AMA." These conceptual assumptions will serve as the basis for the ethical distinctions described later. They are as follows:

1. The medical advice (i.e., recommendation) reflects a measure of absolute rightness.
2. Patients should adhere to medical advice.
3. The AMA discharge is conceptually distinct from the standard discharge process or decision.
4. Patients who do not accept the physician's recommendation to promote the patient's health are behaving oppositionally.

The Ethics of Medical Advice

To better understand AMA discharges, we need a fuller discussion of medical advice, which is arguably central to the practice of medicine. Patients want and expect their physicians to provide them with a medical recommendation, so they can make well-informed choices about their care. Patients report that they don't want their physician to simply provide a list of medical options for them to choose from but rather to provide a recommendation for the best course of action. Physicians are not expected to simply be technical experts on medical options but rather a trusted advisor who can provide needed context for individualizing treatment decisions that fit patient's unique needs. In navigating this sometimes uncertain terrain, the treatment relationship fosters a central alliance where the patient can entrust their care to the physician. This entrustment forms the foundation for high-quality care with health-care decisions that are both medically appropriate and consistent with the patient's individual preferences and needs. The trust also protects patients in ways that are not always obvious to them. A patient's unappreciated cognitive biases may lead them to request care that won't promote their health and well-being. In those cases, physician recommendations can bring to light the need for further consideration and cause patients to alter their choices more in line with their authentic preferences.

Typically, medical advice results from a physician's synthesis of medical science, clinical judgment, and practical experience and is filtered through the physician's professional values. This advice is also affected by decision-making heuristics and their unintended biases (e.g., anchoring, availability, confirmation, etc.) and can be influenced by the physician's personal biases. Although financial conflicts of interest have a recognized potential to bias a wide range of decisions, recent research suggests that non-clinical factors like patient race or socioeconomic status and physician medical specialty or geographic practice area may have a biasing effect on the physician's recommendation and advice-giving process. Therefore, medical advice in reality is most often not an *absolute* truth of rightness but one truth. This advice is subject to reevaluation and reshaping often in response to a number of variables including patient's concerns, values, and preferences and institutional and system factors, among others. In less fraught circumstances (e.g., routine outpatient evaluation), medical advice is widely appreciated to be a well-considered judgment, not precept, and this understanding is reflected in the established practice of obtaining a medical "second opinion." Because the recommendation is still the result of a human enterprise with all its accompanying potential human and system errors, different physicians can come to different, but still "right," conclusions for the patient.

The Role of Power with Advice

Medical advice and decisions about AMA discharges are informed by the power dynamics between patients and physicians. The physician's advice cannot (nor should not) be dissociated from the power of that societal position. In writing about the ethics of medical authority, Howard Brody described the social and technical elements that constitute physician power and how that authority is used to promote essential tenets of professionalism and patient-centered care. The technical elements of power are more easily recognized by both patients and health-care professionals alike. This is the technical knowledge and specialized expertise that health-care professionals possess from their extensive education and training. The technical authority lends them power because it is a specialized brand of knowledge possessed only by physicians, leading to an information asymmetry between the patient and physician.

The social authority is probably felt and wielded more often than it is explicitly acknowledged. This is the institutional power that physicians hold by nature of the profession's established position in society. The professionalization of the practice of medicine has led to its state-sanctioned monopoly for licensed practice and to its authority to self-regulate its practices and its members (e.g., board certification, etc.). Only by completing specific educational and training requirements does the state grant exclusive authority to practice medicine.

Physicians are relied upon to make expert medical determinations that may limit an individual's freedom. In this role, physicians have the authority to commit a patient (i.e., hospitalize against their will) to a psychiatric hospital if in their professional judgment they believe the patient is a danger to themselves or others. They also wield this authority in making official determinations about suitability for certain social services like disability benefits.

This power then, in both its technical and socialized forms and in its implicit and explicit expression, informs the process by which physicians deliberate, make recommendations, and decide about AMA discharges. In its technical form, physicians use their power of specialized knowledge of the benefits of inpatient treatment to persuade patients to remain hospitalized. The informed consent process, which explicitly shares specialized medical information about the discharge decision, is a way to literally share the technical power the physician has over the patient. By providing patients medical information, physicians reduce the knowledge asymmetry and decrease the power differential that may contribute to a conflict. More information leads to more engagement in decisions about care.

The social power that physicians possess as a member of their profession is also used in persuading patients to remain hospitalized. Within the hospital environment, physicians generally represent authority figures, who may not be easily questioned. This power is used to influence patients to pursue behaviors and actions that promote their health.

Shared Decision-Making

Ideally, the eventual plan of care does not necessarily hew narrowly to medical knowledge alone, but rather it reflects a patient-centered consensus between patient and physician. This plan reflects several clinical considerations such as the likelihood, nature, and degree of both harms and benefits, as well as the values, interests, and priorities of the patient. This process of consensus development is contemporarily described as *shared decision-making* (SDM). It is worth reiterating that SDM refers to a *process* designed to meaningfully engage patients in articulating their values and preferences in the context of the available medical evidence and not to a particular decision-making result. Even when carried out fully, this process may result in varying degrees of consensus or, in fact, no consensus between patient and physician.

SDM may still be an aspirational process for some physicians as something short of this is more typical in clinical care. The relative success of SDM is affected by a variety of factors tied to physicians, patients, and health-care system concerns. Beginning with hospitalized patients, they may be at particular risk for not engaging in SDM with their health-care providers. These patients can be poorly situated to receive complex information about their health. Health literacy, emotional state, and physical symptoms can each pose a barrier to acquisition of complex, time-sensitive medical information. Many patients, particularly those with chronic illnesses and frequent hospitalizations, enter the health-care environment with a predisposition toward mistrust or antipathy that often is not without basis. Some patients may struggle with engaging with the physician's advice due to controlling influences such as addictions to substances that compel the patient to leave in order to seek them, some psychiatric illnesses, and compelling responsibilities to others including serious financial hardships. Some patients who seek discharge AMA are, nevertheless, receptive to hearing ways in which the risks associated with premature discharge can be minimized and alternative ways they can seek care in the future. These patients should be deeply engaged.

Similarly, physicians may be unprepared to engage in SDM with hospitalized patients for a variety of reasons. Often, therapeutic relationships between patient and physician are not well developed due to the brevity and often the discontinuity of contact between the principals common in hospital care. Depending on the ability of the physician to engage empathically, some of these patients leave the hospital with elevated levels of emotionality and with rancor.

Physicians do not always effectively inform patients about their condition and full range of treatment options, using medical jargon and euphemisms, and sometimes present subjective information as an objective assessment. System barriers to good physician-led communication include increasing workload, time pressure, computer distractions, and discontinuity or fragmentations of care. These and other factors undercut the development and maintenance of a therapeutic environment and relationship building that supports SDM processes.

Even under ideal conditions of time and adequate skill development, achieving wider adoption of SDM will require broader acceptance of its role in more areas of medical decision-making. SDM is designed to apply to a broad range of "preference-sensitive" health-care decisions, some of which physicians may not believe or are able to apply to inpatient care or discharge planning. Preference-sensitive decisions indicate that a patient's values and preferences are relevant to the ultimate health-care decision. For example, the decision to have a screening mammogram is preference-sensitive because patients have varying tolerances toward risk or for generating information that may not affect meaningful health-care outcomes. If the results of a mammogram are more likely to generate anxiety about cancer (e.g., false-positive finding resulting in a negative tissue biopsy) than it is to generate information that is likely to reduce the patient's risk of dying from cancer, then some patient's may choose to forgo it. In this way, the decision is not one borne entirely of dispassionate medical facts in a vacuum but rather patient's values and preferences about how they wish to make health-care decisions.

Although there is evidence that physicians are willing to engage in SDM for decisions about cancer screening tests (e.g., mammography and prostate-specific antigen testing), there is less evidence that it is regularly applied to discharge planning decisions in the inpatient environment. It is unknown whether this is due to physicians' lack of necessary skills to engage in this process, a belief that decisions about inpatient care should be minimally subject to patient preference, or an unwillingness to practice SDM because of a more time-pressured inpatient environment.

SDM may improve the quality of decisions consistent with a patient's values and preferences, but it will not necessarily produce a consensus between the patient and the physician. Although SDM seeks to optimize patient autonomy and patient's best interest, physicians may still struggle with the inherent tension in this value conflict. Ultimately, resolving it demands a patient-centered perspective that recognizes the patient's role in health-care decisions and its relevance to overall health-care quality. Patient-centered care was defined by the Institute of Medicine in their report, *Crossing the Quality Chasm*, as "providing care that respects and recognizes patients' values and preferences and ensures that those preferences guide all decision making." In this report, the IOM helped to establish that patient-centeredness is as crucial to health-care quality as other recognized factors like equity, effectiveness, timeliness, and safety.

In circumstances when a patient wishes to leave the hospital prior to a safe clinical endpoint, the physician may feel they are not able to responsibly accept the patient's decision because of the high attendant likelihood of harm. Nevertheless, from an ethics perspective, the physician should adopt a non-abandonment, harm reduction stance toward the patient's care. The principle of harm reduction is consistent with the tenets of professionalism because it seeks to balance competing priorities so that the patient can receive the best care they are currently *willing* to accept. Harm reduction attempts to mitigate some of the anticipated patient harms that may result from non-health-promoting behaviors while accepting that patients may continue in those behaviors. Widely accepted, evidence-based harm reduction strategies include nicotine replacement therapy and needle exchange programs. Although some physicians may be uncomfortable with offering suboptimal, harm-reducing recommendations or participating directly in nonconforming medical practice, harm reduction programs like clean needle exchanges have been demonstrated to be effective in improving health outcomes and enhancing continued access to health care.

The value of harm reduction is that physicians focus primarily on the patient's welfare and, where the medical interventions are not likely to cause net or imminent harm, physicians set aside their own reluctance in order to engage patients on their own terms. This stance is consistent with the notion of professionalism in which self-interest is subjugated to professional obligations and patient's interests.

Voluntary Informed Consent

A key ethical concern in discharge AMA is the degree to which patients' decisions are not only informed but the degree to which they are voluntary. By voluntary we mean decisions that the individual would reliably make under similar circumstances and without substantially controlling influences. As part of informed consent, the physician provides the patient with information relevant to the decision to leave the hospital. Then the physician should ensure the patient understands the information because misunderstanding or ignorance undermines the patient's voluntariness. Indeed, the most common reason patients decline inpatient treatment is lack of information. Institutions have an ethical duty to protect and support patients in this regard, and its clinical teams should expend reasonable efforts to identify and to mitigate controlling influences that interfere with the informed consent process, commensurate with reasonably available resources.

Voluntariness is also affected by the content and the quality of the information provided. Multiple studies have demonstrated that physicians believe and disclose to patients that if they leave AMA, their insurance will not pay for the hospitalization. Although the available empirical evidence indicates that payment is not denied by either private or government payers, this oft-provided misinformation about financial penalties undermines patients' ability to make a voluntary choice. Similarly, isolated reports of physicians denying access to otherwise medically indicated discharge services to patients who leave AMA (e.g., transportation, medication) suggest a poorly informed but undeniably coercive attempt to persuade a patient to remain hospitalized. This practice reduces a patient's ability to voluntarily deliberate about his choices for discharge and is a misuse of the physician's social power described earlier.

Patients who leave the hospital abruptly and without an informed consent discussion do not give their clinicians the opportunity to adequately counsel their patients. In these circumstances, the patient has not received or has declined to receive the relevant medical counsel. Here, we make the distinction between patients who leave *against* medical advice and those who leave *without* medical advice. If adequate counseling cannot be achieved for any reason, then the patient should be considered to be discharged *without* medical advice. These scenarios are often referred to colloquially as "elopement." Arguably, these situations are often more frustrating for clinicians who often believe that they did not have fair opportunity to reason with the patient for the patient's benefit.

Patients who leave *against* medical advice have made an informed, and ideally voluntary, decision to decline medical advice for hospitalization. The corollary in AMA discharges to informed consent to treatment is informed withholding of consent. In this case, physicians are obligated to attempt to engage patients in a process of counseling similar to the process used in securing informed consent. AMA discharge counseling should include a discussion of the likelihood of harms of leaving, the likelihood of benefits of remaining hospitalized, the magnitude of each of these, and any medically acceptable alternatives to leaving when they exist, as well as a discussion of the trade-offs inherent in the choices. This process has been alternatively referred to as "informed refusal" or refusal of care after an informed consent discussion.

Do the duties and obligations of the physician differ with respect to patients who leave *against* medical advice as compared to patients who leave *without* medical advice? Physicians' basic duties to patients who leave *without* medical advice are to ensure that hospital resources have been appropriately expended in order to improve the quality of the patient's decision-making and to maximize his or her health, to create and offer a safe as possible discharge plan, and to support the patient in securing post-hospital care. These duties toward patients who leave *without* medical advice continue to exist, although it may be much more difficult for physicians to satisfy these obligations or be accountable for the health outcomes.

Care Venues and Medical Advice

So far in this discussion, we have described patients acting "against medical advice" as a phenomenon particular to the hospital. However, many would recognize that discharge AMA is merely one manifestation of non-concordance between physicians' advice and patients' choices, and that this is common throughout the continuum of clinical care. Situations typically described as AMA differ only in weightiness of consequence from the more ubiquitous instances of non-consensus. The ethical principles do not change, nor do the rights of patients or the obligations of physicians. Decisional discordance occurs in both outpatient and inpatient settings and for clinical scenarios ranging from low-consequence to life-threatening. Nevertheless, the institutional, inpatient setting lends itself to a particular tyranny of the locale. Patients declining medical recommendations take on greater intensity for clinicians in hospitals likely because they have particular control over patients and concerns of clinical and legal liability may amplify these factors. Circumstances may be also charged for patients, albeit in a reciprocal manner, as they commonly experience diminished control, identity, individuality, and autonomy when hospitalized.

Patient nonadherence, although relatively infrequent in the inpatient setting, is an extraordinarily common phenomenon in outpatient clinical care and occurs in office practices, urgent care settings, and infusion centers. For example, patients are non-adherent to antihypertensive medication regimen as much as 30% of the time. In these settings, nonadherence does not typically trigger a formalized administrative response such as the filing of unique forms requiring patient signature. To illustrate, consider an example where an office patient is prescribed a medically indicated cholesterol-lowering medication for hyperlipidemia and on follow-up visit is found to have never started the therapy. The patient's decision to refrain from this medication is by one technical description against medical advice. A typical response by the physician is to re-counsel the patient and document the discussion regarding the patient's nonadherence. Patients in these circumstances are not routinely expected to sign forms attesting to their decision, and physicians do not typically make pronouncements about the patient's insight or decision-making capacity.

To illustrate further, a cancer patient in an infusion center might become symptomatically hypotensive from chemotherapy-induced diarrhea yet declines admonitions by the clinical staff to be admitted to the hospital for treatment. The consequences of nonadherence may be as serious as any inpatient's circumstance, yet as far as what has been published in the literature or what we can discern, there are no parallels to formalized hospital-based AMA discharge practices in infusion centers and no routinely used term to describe this.

Discharge Decisions by Surrogate Decision-Makers

AMA decisions by proxy are more complex and can amplify the ethical challenges of surrogate decision-making. This describes a discharge decision by a patient's authorized decision-maker when the patient lacks decision-making capacity. These challenges involve the nature of the patient-surrogate relationship, the ethical basis for surrogate decisions, and the, respectively, mutually held interests of the patient and surrogate. The clinical features of AMA by surrogate decision-makers differ from patient-directed discharge in that illnesses that sometime fuel discharge AMA, such as substance use disorders, are likely less common of an issue for surrogates than it is for patients. Additionally, differences between the patient-physician relationship and the surrogate-physician relationship may affect the way in which medical advice is received and considered. However, surrogate's experience of AMA discharges may parallel those of patients in that they both may have distrust of the health system, low health literacy, or impairment due to medical or psychiatric illnesses.

This discussion presumes that surrogate's authority to make health-care decisions on behalf of the patient begins *only* after the patient has been determined to have impaired capacity to render decisions about treatment and disposition. Inpatients who lack sufficient decision-making capacity have at least two advocates: their authorized surrogate decision-maker (e.g., a designated health-care agent, next of kin, etc.) and the health professionals who are duty bound to care for the patient. Under what circumstances do surrogates have the ethical authority to remove patients from the hospital AMA and what obligations exist for professionals? Surrogates are morally empowered to make decisions on behalf of patients consistent with the patient's explicit or inferred wishes (i.e., substituted judgment). If the patient's wishes are not known, surrogates are minimally charged with making decisions that they believe serves the patient's best interests. Under these criteria for surrogate decision-making, a surrogates' removal of a patient from the hospital AMA would have to be based on the surrogates' considered assessment that the patient would not have wanted inpatient medical treatment plan under these circumstances or that, in balancing the benefits and burdens of the hospitalization, leaving the hospital now would be more beneficial to the patient than remaining (i.e., in his best interest). If the surrogate's plan is to remove the patient to home, then in order to satisfy the best interest standard, medical interventions in the hospital would have to be sufficiently substandard to render home-based care, outpatient follow-up, or no care at home less harmful than the medical care provided in the hospital. Of course, this determination rests upon the principle that surrogates may have differing conceptions from physicians of what constitutes benefit and harm for the patient. In general, surrogates are given a wide scope of authority for making these determinations.

Conclusion

AMA discharges are both clinically and ethically challenging. Physicians working to balance their dual obligations to respect patient's autonomy to make decisions consistent with their own values, wishes, and desires can conflict with the physician's other obligations to provide the patient with care believed to be in the patient's best interest. Applying harm reduction and shared decision-making actions in discharge planning provides guiding principles for the physician wishing to negotiate these competing values and work more productively with patients.

Suggested Reading

1. Alfandre D. Reconsidering against medical advice discharges: embracing patient-centeredness to promote high quality care and a renewed research agenda. J Gen Intern Med. 2013;28(12):1657–62. https://doi.org/10.1007/s11606-013-2540-z. Epub 2013 Jul
2. Alfandre D. Clinical recommendations in medical practice – a proposed framework for reducing bias and improving decision quality. J Clin Ethics. 2016;27(1):21–7.
3. Beauchamp TL, Childress JF. Principles of biomedical ethics. 7th ed. New York: Oxford University Press; 2012. p. 137–8.
4. Berger JT. Discharge against medical advice: ethical considerations and professional obligations. J Hosp Med. 2008;3(5):403–8. https://doi.org/10.1002/jhm.362.
5. Berger JT, DeRenzo EG, Schwartz J. Surrogate decision making: reconciling ethical theory and clinical practice. Ann Intern Med. 2008;149:48–53.
6. Brody H. The healer's power. New Haven: Yale University Press; 1993.
7. Fischer MA, Stedman MR, Lii J, Vogeli C, Shrank WH, Brookhart MA, Weissman JS. Primary medication non-adherence: analysis of 195,930 electronic prescriptions. J Gen Intern Med. 2010;25(4):284–90.
8. Lekas HM, Alfandre D, Gordon P, Harwood K, Yin MT. The role of patient-provider interactions: using an accounts framework to explain hospital discharges against medical advice. Soc Sci Med. 2016;156:106–13. https://doi.org/10.1016/j.socscimed.2016.03.018. Epub 2016 Mar 15
9. Tollen WB. Irregular discharge: the problem of hospitalization of the tuberculous. Public Health Rep. 1948;63(45):1441–73.
10. Windish DM, Ratanawongsa N. Providers' perceptions of relationships and professional roles when caring for patients who leave the hospital against medical advice. J Gen Intern Med. 2008;23:1698.

Chapter 5
Reframing the Phenomenon of Discharges Against Medical Advice: A Sociologist's Perspective

Helen-Maria Lekas

Introduction

When a patient leaves the hospital before the treating provider's recommendation, the discharge is deemed against medical advice (AMA). In the USA, approximately 500,000 or 2% of all annual hospital discharges occur against medical advice [1, 2]. The low prevalence of AMA events seems to have fostered the belief that their contribution to human suffering and healthcare costs is limited and that these events are epidemiologically trivial. The lack of research and interventions on this topic also signal that the phenomenon of leaving the hospital AMA is considered of little public health significance.

However, beyond the numerical rarity of AMA discharges, a review of the literature reveals several salient points that suggest the need to revisit our assessment of this phenomenon. First, studies have substantiated that the highest rates of AMA events occur among the most psychosocially vulnerable patients affected by potentially stigmatizing conditions, that is, patients with mental illness, substance use disorder, and/or infected with the human immunodeficiency virus (HIV) [3, 4]. Second, in terms of sociodemographic characteristics, male gender, younger age, poverty or low socioeconomic status (SES), and being uninsured or insured by Medicaid have been associated with leaving the hospital AMA [1, 5]. Although it is not unequivocal, belonging to a racial/ethnic minority group has also been associated with AMA discharge in several studies [2, 4–6]. Third, a discharge AMA is a predictor of a subsequent AMA discharge from the hospital. Also, compared to patients conventionally discharged, patients who leave the hospital AMA experience

H. -M. Lekas (✉)
Nathan Kline Institute for Psychiatric Research, Division of Social Solutions and Social Research, Orangeburg, NY 10962, USA

Department of Sociomedical Sciences, Mailman School of Public Health, Columbia University Medical Center, New York, NY, USA
e-mail: helen-maria.lekas@nki.rfmh.org

© Springer International Publishing AG, part of Springer Nature 2018
D. Alfandre (ed.), *Against-Medical-Advice Discharges from the Hospital*,
https://doi.org/10.1007/978-3-319-75130-6_5

higher rates of morbidity and mortality [1, 4]. Therefore, AMA events tend to involve primarily psychosocially marginalized and stigmatized patients and to expose them to severe, adverse health and healthcare utilization consequences, including misuse of services and preventable deaths. These findings suggest that AMA discharges most likely constitute one of the mechanisms that produce and reproduce health disparities.

Three additional features of the literature also hint at the need to reconsider the research and public health significance of AMA events. First, the overwhelming majority of studies identify the characteristics of patients who leave AMA and are based on quantitative retrospective analyses of medical records. Empirical studies that collect data directly from patients or content analyses of records are scarce. Consequently, we know very little about what actually happens when patients decide to leave a hospital AMA, including the patients' reasons for doing so. The limitations of a body of literature based primarily on medical records data (e.g., records are composed by providers often to fulfill institutional mandates) have been largely overlooked. Second, studies that include data on the providers' perspectives and experiences related to AMA events are almost absent. Yet, numerous editorials and commentaries written by clinicians reveal that they contend with several practical and ethical challenges related to AMA discharges. An AMA event by default includes one or more treating providers who try to avert the patient's premature departure. Therefore, providers' perspectives and experiences are a critical component of the AMA phenomenon. Third, with the exception of a few studies that include hospital-level variables in their AMA analysis (e.g., hospital size; ownership such as public, private, not-for-profit; or geographical location) [2, 6–9], most researchers do not consider the role of the institutional setting in AMA events. AMA events do not occur in an institutional vacuum but instead are influenced by the policies, regulations, and often tacit routines of hospitals. All of the aforementioned gaps in the literature suggest that our understanding of AMA discharges and their potential role in health disparities is limited.

In this chapter, I revisit the phenomenon of AMA discharge and propose three constructs, "habitus," "institutional agency," and "strategic research event," as interpretative tools that will enable a reconceptualization of the phenomenon of leaving the hospital AMA and a reevaluation of its epidemiological and public health significance. Further, I will propose that engaging in "institutional ethnography" has the potential to elicit comprehensive data on AMA discharges that can contribute to the design of much-needed interventions.

Concepts as Hermeneutic Tools

It is useful to provide the definitions of the concepts mentioned above before using them in a critical review of the AMA literature. The first concept, *habitus*, pertains to both patients and providers interacting and communicating around an AMA event. To address a core sociological question, what accounts for social patterns and regularities in human behavior, Pierre Bourdieu coined the term habitus to refer to individuals' durable dispositions to view the world, assess it, and act in certain ways [10, 11]. He posited that habitus emerges at the intersection of social structure and individual agency. Specifically, an individual's place in the social structure determines his/her life opportunities or chances, whereas agency determines one's life choices. Opportunities or lack thereof enhance or constrain an individual's range of choices. The interplay between choices and opportunities shapes an individual's habitus. Habitus motivates behavior, and overtime, behavior crystalizes into a lifestyle. A unique feature of habitus is that often it operates mechanically when motivating behavior, instead of thoughtfully. That is, habitus generates behavior almost through an unconscious process, and this tends to reproduce the same behavior. Moreover, because of its social origin, individuals who occupy a similar place in the social structure (e.g., belong to the same social class, racial group, or professional group) tend to develop similar habitus, behaviors, and lifestyle. Both patients and providers bring to the AMA event their own habitus that informs their actions that have the potential to avert or to produce an AMA discharge. Given the psychosocial vulnerability of patients most likely to leave the hospital AMA and the providers' medical authority, I propose using the concept of habitus to shed light on the patient-provider interactions and communication processes that result in AMA discharges.

The second concept of *institutional agency* refers to the fact that organizations and systems, like individuals, engage in differentiating practices, that is, they have agency. This agentic feature becomes apparent in the tasks and practices of service providers, of administrators that enforce rules and regulations, and of policymakers that generate macro-level policies that frame institutional operations. As an outcome of having agency, institutions do not provide equitable services or resources to all clients or patients with whom they interface but instead tend to favor those higher up in the social structure. Attributing agency to institutions and recognizing that the services they provide differentially benefit service recipients suggest a mechanism that produces inequities. The concept of institutional agency has been used by Lutfey and Freese to explain how patients' characteristics (e.g., social class, race, ethnicity, or gender) tend to elicit different responses from the same healthcare institutions and providers and how this results in health disparities [12, 13]. AMA events unfold in the institutional setting of the hospital, and therefore, the hospital's agency – expressed in routine practices, regulations, and policies – determines both the experiences of providers attempting to care for patients and of patients exercising their right to leave. Therefore, using the construct of institutional agency has the potential to elicit data that contextualize the actions taken and constraints faced by both providers and patients that ultimately shape an AMA event.

The sociological approach of *institutional ethnography* was developed by Dorothy Smith and her colleagues [14–16]. This ethnographic approach highlights the importance of analyzing the organizational artifacts generated by service providers (e.g., medical records, number of syringes used on a hospital floor, or written discharge instructions given to patients) while also examining their everyday activities and those of the people they serve. Through observation and in-depth interviewing, institutional ethnographers understand the routine tasks and experiences of service providers and service recipients. However, they also collect seemingly mundane institutional artifacts, such as memoranda on staff communication or schedule of staff meetings and case conferencing, and by analyzing their meaning better reveal the workings of an institution. The textual analysis of these artifacts reveals a hospital's management style, regulations, explicit strategies, or tacit ways of operating. These institutional features, in turn, are determined by and therefore reflect the macro sociocultural context (e.g., negative stereotypes assigned to drug use or to patients receiving public assistance). Consequently, institutional ethnography is a method of eliciting institutional agency and contextualizing the experiences of both service providers and recipients and, therefore, is well suited for examining AMA events.

The fourth concept of *strategic research event (SRE)* was coined by Robert Merton [17] to explain the scientific practice of selecting to investigate a particular event that reveals a phenomenon with such clarity that it promotes the understanding of fundamental issues related to this phenomenon, contributes to relevant theory, or reveals new related questions. That is, the scientific utility of a SRE extends beyond the understanding of the particular event examined, and this increases its epistemic value. Specifically, a SRE is an empirical event that "...exhibits the phenomena to be explained or interpreted to such advantage and in such accessible form that it enables the fruitful investigation of previously stubborn problems and the discovery of new problems for fruitful inquiry" (p. 11). I propose that the AMA discharge phenomenon is a SRE because it brings in sharp focus the forces that undermine the patient-provider relationship and, moreover, when the patient is already involved in the medical care system and sick enough to require hospitalization. Further, the setting of the hospital provides the opportunity to examine this relationship in context and, thus, shed light on the institutional features that influence patient-provider interactions.

In the sections that follow, I review the AMA literature using the concepts defined above with the goal of substantiating that AMA events contribute to health disparities and enhance the understanding of patient-centered care and, therefore, have high public health significance. As the reader will recognize, most of the empirical literature on AMA focuses on patients. This can be interpreted as an indication that the field is attributing the AMA discharge primarily to the patient. My goal is by the end of this chapter to convince the reader that AMA events are the outcome of patient-provider interactions that are located in and influenced by the institutional setting of the hospital. Moreover, I aim to define AMA events as strategic research events (SREs) that reveal healthcare processes that contribute to health disparities and, thus, enhance the public health significance of the phenomenon of AMA discharges.

Discharge AMA: Where the Patient Habitus and the Provider Habitus Interface

Patient Habitus from the Margins, a Habitus Informed by Structure

Even a cursory review of the literature on leaving the hospital AMA reveals that the occurrence of this type of discharge is not equally distributed among the different patient groups. In terms of medical diagnosis, individuals with psychiatric illness, substance use disorder (including alcohol), and HIV have the highest rates of AMA discharges, 6–54%, 20–50%, and 10–30%, respectively, across studies [3, 4, 18, 19]. The features shared by these three medical conditions are that they are chronic, they are difficult to manage, and they tend to cluster as comorbidities. As a result, patients with a substance use disorder (SUD) are at increased odds of being HIV infected and/or have a psychiatric diagnosis. Moreover, all three conditions tend to confer stigma to the sufferers. Acquiring HIV and/or a substance use disorder (SUD) are often seen as outcomes of moral and behavioral irresponsibility, and this contributes to their stigmatizing status [20, 21]. Although the attribution of psychiatric illness to the lack of personal will or moral courage has been debunked, it remains a highly stigmatizing condition primarily because of its association with dangerous, seemingly irrational, and unpredictable behavior [22]. Patients with these conditions very likely have been stigmatized by others post disclosure of their diagnosis and often prior to becoming hospitalized. As substantiated by the stigma literature, stigmatization of these patients discredits and, more importantly, excludes them from housing, employment, educational, and social engagement opportunities that also limit their choices. Stigma effectively traps them at the lower rungs of the socioeconomic status (SES) hierarchy by depriving them of basic life opportunities [23–26]. Because of these exclusionary experiences, I suggest that these patient populations tend to develop a disposition of being socially disenfranchised, an alienated habitus that often motivates them to hide, withdraw, or flee to avoid exposure to stigmatizing or seemingly stigmatizing behavior (e.g., delay in receiving test results or inadequate management of pain associated with withdrawal from drugs). This *habitus from the margins*, as I propose we call it, has the potential to influence their behavior and interactions in the hospital and can contribute to leaving the hospital AMA.

Indications of this habitus from the margins can also be found in the studies that have identified the patient sociodemographic characteristics that predict AMA discharge, that is, being male, young in age, uninsured or Medicaid insured, and poor or of low socioeconomic status (SES). Some studies have also demonstrated that racial or ethnic minority status also increases the likelihood of AMA discharge, while other studies indicate that when controlling for low SES, the effect of race and ethnicity disappears. These characteristics compose the profile of a patient that has developed a habitus shaped by the limited opportunities and choices available in the low rungs of the SES hierarchy. Also, given his male gender, young age, and insurance status, most likely he has had limited experience with the healthcare system and providers. The likelihood that, prior to his hospitalization, he will have been invited to establish a therapeutic alliance with a healthcare provider, develop trust, and learn to prioritize his health is very slim. Instead, his habitus will have been shaped by being deprived of opportunities (e.g., education, jobs), subjected to different forms of social control (e.g., foster care, police harassment), and mostly, by engaging in activities to make ends meet. All this shapes his approach to interacting with social institutions and individuals that have authority, including medical. Therefore, his behavior in the hospital likely will be motivated by a habitus from the margins that is not conducive to establishing a good patient-provider relationship and equates autonomy with the right to remove oneself from a situation that he perceives as restrictive or even punitive. This patient disposition can contribute to an AMA discharge.

In reviewing the literature, I identified some empirical findings that support this notion that in AMA events, a patient habitus from the margins might be operating. First, several studies have demonstrated that a prior AMA discharge predicts a subsequent such discharge [3–5, 7, 27, 28]. For instance, Alfandre and colleagues [27] using records data from a large New York City hospital found that in 2012–2013, among HIV-infected inpatients, more than one fourth of AMA discharges occurred among patients with multiple AMA discharges. This percentage rose to 33% for inpatients with alcohol-related disorders. A history of leaving the hospital AMA has been identified as an AMA discharge risk factor, and in one study, it was deemed as red-flag patient behavior raising provider concern about patient drug seeking [29]. The same group of researchers also linked a history of leaving the hospital AMA with lower patient trust in the medical profession, thus suggesting that AMA events generate and signal both provider and patient distrust [30]. More than two decades ago, Jeremiah and colleagues [28] posited that the association between prior and subsequent AMA discharge "…suggests a pattern of behavior that adds to our understanding of the AMA phenomenon" (p. 405). I concur and propose to conceptualize this pattern of behavior as the outcome of a habitus from the margins that accounts for why patients engage with the healthcare system and providers in a tenuous manner so that almost any reason can be used to justify their leaving the hospital AMA, as discussed next.

The second set of findings that point to a particular patient habitus refers to the reported or inferred reasons for leaving the hospital AMA. The few studies that have examined patients' reasons for AMA discharge revealed that patients reported a variety of reasons for leaving the hospital, that patient and provider assessments of the patient's health often diverge, and that a significant minority of patients do not provide any reason for leaving or leave without informing hospital staff. Across studies, patients offered different explanations for their departure from the hospital, including having to attend to personal or family obligations, financial matters, job commitments, housing issues, feeling better or feeling bored, wanting to use drugs or alcohol, and being dissatisfied with medical care [28, 31, 32]. Many of these reasons were not health related but stemmed from patients' everyday life challenges and responsibilities. For instance, two studies noted that the rates of AMA discharges increased on dates when public assistance checks were issued and concluded that this benefit motivated patients' premature departures [3, 18]. I suggest that the habitus of low SES patients that is shaped by daily stressors and hardships related to lack of opportunities tends to prioritize meeting one's survival needs instead of one's health. This lifestyle is also associated with interacting only sporadically with healthcare providers and the system, typically around a health crisis. Indeed, a study by Jeremiah and colleagues [28] indicated that not having a primary physician was significantly associated with leaving AMA. From the patients' perspective and experience that are instilled in their habitus, faced with the dilemma of staying and attending to their health or leaving to attend to their life challenges (e.g., losing one's job, cash benefits, or food stamps), I propose that departing the hospital AMA might make good sense.

Patients who attributed their premature departure from the hospital to dissatisfaction with care mentioned disagreements with providers about the need for tests, about the management of addiction and withdrawal-related symptoms (e.g., pain), or about the severity of their medical condition. Indeed, a study that assessed the concordance/discordance between patient and provider evaluation of the appropriateness of the patients' hospital stay found that there was little or no agreement on the reasons for the hospital stay and, moreover, that providers were not cognizant of the patients' views [33]. Feeling discredited or disrespected by providers was another feature of dissatisfaction with care. This was most commonly reported by patients with a substance use disorder [34] but was also found in non-substance-using samples [28, 32]. It is significant that in one study that focused on patients that left AMA from the emergency department (ED) after their medical evaluation had begun, some patients were disinclined to return because they were concerned about hospital staff stigmatization [35]. Specifically, among those who did not access medical care within three days as instructed, 20% shared that feeling embarrassed for having left AMA and fearing provider "derision" prevented them from returning to the ED. This finding supports the point made above that one aspect of the habitus of patients leaving the hospital AMA probably is the motivation or tendency to avoid exposure to provider stigmatization. This inference can also be gleaned by the finding that many patients do not provide a reason for their premature departure from the hospital while some leave without informing the staff (an event hospital staff euphemistically calls "elopement"). For instance, in a study by Baptist and colleagues [4], 42.7% of patients reported no reason for leaving AMA, and 15.3% left without informing the hospital staff. In our content analysis of the AMA notes included in patient records, for 30% of the HIV-infected inpatients, we could not infer a reason for leaving AMA because the patient had not offered one or had absconded [36]. Moreover, we found that some patients reported more socially acceptable reasons for leaving AMA (e.g., to take care of one's grandchildren or to avoid being evicted) as excuses or justifications for wanting to prematurely leave, an action they recognized was untoward [36]. These findings raise the important question of whether patients motivated by their habitus from the margins refrain from sharing the actual reasons for wanting to leave with hospital staff fearing a negative response, including being delegitimized. Patients concealing or misrepresenting their true motives for wanting to be discharged detracts from the likelihood that providers will offer them the appropriate support (e.g., adequately managing addiction-related pain) and successfully address their concerns (e.g., discussing patient fear of test results). These missed opportunities for provision of patient-centered care erode the quality of patient-provider relationships, thus reproducing patients' habitus from the margins.

My proposal to use the construct of patient habitus from the margins as a heuristic device to examine the literature is not meant to suggest that I attribute AMA events primarily to patients. An AMA discharge is the outcome of a patient-provider interaction, and therefore, to understand it more fully, I next examine the providers' habitus.

Provider Habitus: An Amalgam of Uncertainty and Authority, an Opportunity for Patient-Centered Care

Given the lack of provider studies, I will assemble the provider habitus related to AMA discharges from editorials and commentaries and the few available empirical studies. When healthcare providers, physicians for the most part, write about their perceptions and experiences related to AMA events, it clearly emerges that they consider these events highly distressing and frustrating [37–41]. These reactions are often caused by the dissonance providers experience from wanting to respect the patient's right to autonomy and self-determination while also wanting to ensure the patient receives optimal care. A core feature of providers' habitus is their medical expertise that motivates them to prioritize the patient's health and, therefore, encourage or persuade the patient to remain in the hospital. The patient's decision to leave AMA tends to challenge this aspect of the providers' habitus. The impact of this process of challenging is discussed below.

Provider frustration is further amplified by the lack of standards regarding the designation of a discharge as AMA and by an ambiguous determination of its legal significance. There is also lack of clarity on whether an AMA discharge form signed by the patient gives providers full legal protection from a medical malpractice suit. For instance, in their review of the literature and discussion of the legal protections an AMA discharge can confer, Levy and colleagues [42] concluded that "A properly executed and documented AMA form can provide significant protection from liability risk" (p. 520). However, in their review of malpractice suits, Devitt and colleagues [40] cautioned physicians and hospitals that if patients experience adverse consequences post discharge, the AMA discharge forms patients signed "… are meaningless and have no legal protection value" (p. 902). This ambiguity regarding the legal significance of a signed AMA form might motivate providers to strongly urge, even pressure, patients to sign it prior to their departure, thus eroding the patient-provider communication and interaction that are already challenged by the impending premature discharge. In the AMA discharge notes we analyzed, the authors (i.e., physicians, nurses, or social workers) routinely reported whether the discharge note was signed by the patient or not, and this suggested that they assigned some significance to this fact [36]. We also recognized that when the staff member writing the AMA note was a provider in the lower rungs of the hospital hierarchy (e.g., a resident or a nurse), he or she tended to call upon other staff or upon a provider higher in the hierarchy (e.g., an attending) to also sign the form in an effort to share responsibility for the AMA event with their colleagues. Therefore, providers seem to assign some legally protective value to these signatures, at minimum from institutional blame. Actually, AMA forms across different hospitals typically include a place for both patient and provider(s) to sign despite the lack of a clear rationale for including these signatures [43].

Another aspect of the AMA event that amplifies providers' apprehension and uncertainty is that many seem to be under the erroneous impression that insurance companies do not cover the hospitalization cost when a patient leaves AMA and share this misinformation with their patients to convince them to stay [43]. In a study by Schaefer and colleagues [44], 70.6% of residents and 51.2% of attending physicians reported that they often or always communicate to their patients that their insurance will not cover their hospital expenses if they leave AMA. Most but not all of these providers considered this statement accurate (i.e., 68% of the residents and 43.9% of the attending physicians). Therefore, some providers seem to misinform patients about this issue of financial responsibility to dissuade them from leaving prematurely. Despite these providers' good intention to protect the patients' health, fabricating a barrier to convince patients to stay in the hospital goes against the principles of patient-centered care and undermines patient trust of providers and healthcare institutions. Moreover, lack of patient trust is a feature of their habitus from the margins, and therefore, misinforming the patient about an aspect of their care has the potential to reproduce this type of habitus and, thus, promote AMA events. However, the decision of some providers to misinform patients also indicates the extent of provider frustration and the lack of alternative strategies to keep patients in the hospital. Providers who believe that insurance plans do not cover the cost associated with a hospitalization that ended in an AMA discharge might perceive averting such a discharge as their institutional duty, and consequently, failing to do so can generate apprehension that also infuses their habitus. All of the aforementioned ambiguities regarding the AMA discharge process generate provider distress and uncertainty about best practices in such instances. I suggest that this uncertainty likely challenges providers' habitus of expertise and authority that has been constructed through their professional training, practice, and the status society and culture assign to the medical profession. As discussed later, the hospital's institutional agency, through rules and policies, also supports provider authority, but this does not seem to avert AMA events.

Indicators that provider experiences associated with AMA events have an effect on their habitus are also provided by the few available empirical studies. Specifically, I identified two qualitative studies [32, 45] that have explored in-depth providers' perceptions, feelings, and actions associated with AMA events. One study included nurses and physicians (and patients) and used a focus group method [32]. The other study focused on physicians and was based on qualitative interviews [45]. Across both studies, providers indicated that patients who decided to leave AMA often lacked understanding of their medical condition and its severity. Motivated by their habitus as medical experts, providers also reported that they tried to explain the health threats and the importance of remaining in the hospital to the patients, but this did not suffice to change the patients' decision. As our content analysis of AMA discharge notes also revealed, the exact medical information and health risks that a premature discharge posed to patients were typically mentioned by providers in their attempt to dissuade patients from leaving [36]. Providers also wrote in the AMA note that they asked the patient to reiterate these risks and dangers to ensure that they understood what was at stake. Nevertheless, these attempts to inform patients about the risk of an AMA discharge did not seem to deter them from departing. As discussed in the patient habitus section, patients often prioritize their personal or family obligations instead of their health and, moreover, evaluate their health differently than providers, and both these dispositions can motivate them to leave the hospital. Indeed, providers have recognized this tension between their patients' understanding and their own views of what is best for the patient. For instance, Berger [39] in a review of the professional and ethical dilemmas raised by AMA discharges suggested that "…patients tend to make decisions based on values and broader interests whereas physicians tend to emphasize more circumscribed medical goals" (p. 404). Consequently, patients and providers use different variables to assess the need for inpatient care. In a study examining the appropriateness of hospital stay from both patient and provider perspective, Rentsch [33] concluded "Patients and health care professionals have a completely unrelated perception of the utility of any given day of hospitalization, and agree little about the reasons justifying a given hospital stay" (p. 575). I suggest we conceptualize this divergence in views as the outcome of the patient's habitus from the margins that prioritizes addressing the challenges of life outside the hospital walls and the provider's habitus that prioritizes the patient's health strictly defined according to the biomedical model. Moreover, I propose that the providers' unsuccessful attempts to convince patients to stay can challenge the providers' self-confidence and habitus of authority that is already challenged by the institutional and legal ambiguities surrounding the AMA discharge process. Our analysis of the AMA discharge notes revealed that the providers authoring these notes (i.e., physicians, nurses, or social workers) at times provided excuses or justifications for failing to keep the patient in the hospital despite their best efforts. In these instances, providers recognized the limitations of their medical expertise and authority [36].

Another significant finding that emerged from the two qualitative studies I have been discussing [32, 45] was that providers suspected that some patients were not forthcoming about the real reasons for wanting to leave and this contributed to provider suspicion that these patients were drug seeking and were manipulating the providers and the hospital. Indeed, lack of trust regarding patients that complain about inadequate pain management or are known to have substance use disorder (SUD) is a feature of provider AMA-related habitus. Provider distrust of patients they label as substance users is a robust finding in the AMA literature and the substance use literature [34, 46–48]. For instance, Haywood and colleagues [29] identified a host of patient behaviors and statuses providers associated with unnecessarily or inappropriately drug seeking among patients with sickle cell disease that causes intense and difficult-to-control pain. Among other behaviors, they found that having a history of signing out AMA and a history of disputes with staff (that often precede an AMA discharge) were among patient characteristics that providers associated with drug seeking and, consequently, made them uneasy. I suggest that labeling these two aspects of patient history as problematic introduces distrust in the provider habitus toward such patients and can make them hypervigilant about potential drug abuse. These conditions, in turn, have the potential to sabotage the patient-provider relationship. By leading to a subsequent AMA discharge, these conditions can generate the dynamic of a self-fulfilling prophesy that accounts for the higher rates of AMA discharges among patients with SUD and related comorbidities (i.e., HIV or psychiatric diagnoses) and also patients with prior AMA events. Moreover, as discussed in the patient habitus section, patients who leave AMA are well aware that some providers approach them with suspicion and label them as difficult-to-manage patients. Especially patients with SUD expect that most providers will stigmatize them, discredit their health complaints, and inadequately manage their symptoms, including underregulating their pain [34, 47, 48]. Therefore, leaving to avoid provider stigmatization and to find relief of one's symptoms using street drugs might make good sense to these patients [34]. In an ethnographic study that unfolded in a hospital and included inpatient physicians and their patients who injected drugs or used crack cocaine, Merrill and colleagues [47] identified a vicious cycle of mistrust between providers and patients generated by the former's concern about being deceived and the latter's fear of being mistreated. This reciprocal lack of trust affected the quality of care providers offered and patients received. The authors concluded "Prior experiences of the exceptionally difficult drug user or of the seemingly abusive and stigmatizing physician powerfully influence subsequent interactions" (p. 331). Similarly, in our analysis of the AMA notes, providers placed the patients' expressed reasons for wanting to leave in quotation marks (" ") to denote that they discredited these reasons as misrepresentations of the truth [36]. Some providers explicitly wrote in the note that the real reason why patients wanted to leave was to engage in substance use, and some providers even shared this suspicion with the patients. The patient-provider dynamic, fostered by the interface between patient habitus from the margins and provider AMA-related habitus (i.e., a mixture of suspicion, concern about being deceived, and medical expertise and authority), can account for why patients with psychiatric diagnoses, SUD, and/or HIV have the highest AMA discharge rates.

However, the two aforementioned qualitative studies and our own work have also demonstrated that providers understood the different emotions and non-health-related concerns patients might have had (e.g., competing responsibilities, fear or frustration with waiting time) that motivated them to leave the hospital. Despite their efforts to show empathy to the patient, providers recognized that communication with patients that left AMA was suboptimal. Insufficient communication with patients and the lack of trust providers often experience around AMA events can

explain the finding that such events challenged providers' self-assessment and professional presentation of self [45]. Specifically, providers indicated that their interactions with patients discharged AMA generated some self-doubt in their ability as
medical providers, uncertainty on whether and how to offer ancillary resources to
patients (e.g., social services), and regret for missing the opportunity to engage with
patients earlier and more effectively. These emotions and perceptions motivated
them to reconsider their professional role and responsibilities toward patients. I suggest we conceptualize these experiences that cause providers to reconsider their
interactions with and approach toward patients as challenges to their professional
habitus that generate an amalgam of uncertainty and authority. By infusing some
uncertainty in the provider habitus of expertise and confidence, AMA events can
create the opportunity to enhance provider humility, thus contributing to patient-
centered care. Specifically, the foundation for a good patient-provider relationship
can be established, if patients recognize the providers' humility and suspend their
own mistrust and fear of stigmatization. Paradoxically, defining AMA events as the
outcome of the interplay between provider habitus and patient habitus can reveal
how providers can practice patient-centered medicine with patients at risk of leaving AMA *because of* and *not despite* these patients' habitus from the margins. This
transformation, however, also depends on the institutional setting of the hospital
within which AMA events and the patient-provider interactions unfold, and therefore, I examine this topic next.

Contextualizing the AMA Event: The Role of Institutional Agency

The institutional setting, that is, the hospital where patient-provider interactions and
AMA events take place, undoubtedly has an impact on these events. This fact has
been increasingly recognized by researchers, and in the past decade, hospital-level
variables have been added to some of the AMA analyses that are based on large
datasets. Hospital size (defined by number of beds as large, medium, or small),
hospital ownership (i.e., public/government funded, private, or not-for-profit), location (urban vs. non-urban/rural), region (Northeast, Midwest, South, and West), and
teaching status are the variables most often included in studies [2, 6–9]. Similar data
patterns have emerged across studies that enhance the prediction of AMA discharges
and promote the discussion of AMA events as contributors to health disparities.
Specifically, it has been substantiated that urban hospitals, hospitals of medium or
large size, or those located in the Northeast had higher odds of patients leaving
AMA, whereas in teaching hospitals and in not-for-profit hospitals, the odds of an
AMA discharge were lower [2, 6, 8, 9]. In addition, Franks and colleagues [6] found
that hospitals with a greater proportion of racial/ethnic minority patients and patients
with Medicaid were at a higher risk of discharging patients AMA. Moreover, when
adjusting for hospital characteristics, the higher rates of AMA discharges among

Black patients disappeared. The researchers concluded that therefore, the higher rates of AMA events among Black patients and Hispanic patients might be associated with their admission to hospitals with higher AMA rates. These findings reveal a vulnerability to AMA events at the institutional level that can be presenting as patient-level factors. Certainly, the interplay between individual- and hospital-level factors requires further clarification. For instance, examining hospital-related variables could meaningfully contribute to the current debate on whether non-White race/ethnicity is a predictor of AMA. However, most studies have not attempted to disentangle individual- from hospital-level factors despite recognizing the need to do so. Consequently, researchers have mostly engaged in conjecture and proposed that, for instance, in larger-size hospitals, provider attentiveness is probably lower and this increases the rate of AMA discharges, whereas in rural hospitals higher familiarity and trust between patients and providers likely contribute to lower AMA rates [8]. Trying to explain why hospitals located in urban areas or in the Northeast or those classified as for profit have increased odds to discharge patients AMA is more challenging [6, 7]. Researchers have recognized that hospital-level data are imperative in understanding and addressing the discharge AMA phenomenon. As Tawk and colleagues [9] concluded, "Knowing that factors such as insurance, hospital ownership, region and hospital size could influence AMA discharges could be used as a point of departure for quality improvement efforts" (p. 130). I concur and further propose that to design effective interventions and programs to avert AMA discharges, we also need to understand the role of the hospital as an institution that is nested in the larger, sociocultural context and that, in turn, provides the context for the patient-provider interactions that can lead to AMA events.

Specifically, I propose to conceptualize the hospital as an institutional entity that has agency, that is, discretionary power, and, therefore, can differentially benefit patients [13]. To account for health disparities, research has focused on identifying barriers to accessing medical care. Although significant, access to care is only the first step. The experiences patients have once they engage with the healthcare system directly influence their retention in care and health outcomes [12]. Attributing agency to hospitals enables us to recognize that the types and quality of care (e.g., being placed in a room with other sicker patients or waiting a long time for test results), interactions with providers (e.g., overextended providers not taking the time to explain test results or physicians underregulating pain because of lack of expertise in addiction medicine), and therefore, health benefits patients get from staying in the hospital can vary by institution. Institutional agency connotes that discrepancies in the medical benefits patients experience depend on institutional characteristics above and beyond patient habitus and provider habitus. By institutional characteristics, I refer to the hospital-level variables considered in quantitative analyses and discussed above but also other factors that determine the explicit and implicit workings of the hospital. For instance, patient-to-provider ratio can translate into provider time pressure and cognitive load that, in turn, impact the patient-provider interactions and can contribute to patient dissatisfaction and decision to leave AMA. Availability of ancillary services, such as patient navigators, language translators, or health educators, generates the likelihood that patients will feel supported and decide to adhere to providers' suggestion to stay in the hospital. Whether a hospital fosters a team-based vs. a hierarchical approach to care can also inform how providers practice and how patients perceive and evaluate their hospital stay (e.g., less experienced providers being able to consult with their supervisors on how to interpret ambiguous test results vs. hospital regulations dictating that attending physicians but not nurses who interact with patients longer have the authority to sign an AMA form). Therefore, it is important to also consider implicit features of the hospital's institutional agency that cannot be quantified and systematically collected from all hospitals and, thus, are not included in the American Hospital Association or the National Inpatient Sample, databases used by the studies above that identified the association of hospital-level variables with AMA discharges.

Without using the term institutional agency, a small body of literature is emerging that reveals the hospital as a "risk environment" for inpatients with substance use disorder [34, 48]. For instance, McNeil and colleagues [34] substantiated that abstinence-only drug policies combined with hospital features that do not prioritize adequate management of withdrawal symptoms or in-hospital supervised drug consumption harms patients with substance use disorder (SUD). Specifically, they indicate that hospital characteristics promote in-hospital unsafe drug use and/or AMA discharges thus endangering the health of patients with SUD. These researchers used the term "contextual forces" to account for institutional agency when they referred to several explicit and implicit hospital features that indirectly deem and treat patients with SUD worse than seemingly non-drug-using patients. For instance, hospital policies that prevent the provision of methadone maintenance treatment on premises or the informal practice of placing patients with SUD under closer surveillance are manifestations of the hospital's discretionary power. Ti and colleagues [48] that also identified the hospital as a "risk environment" for persons with SUD concluded that "...the existence of required structure and rules" in a hospital can contribute to these patients leaving AMA. Finally, an ethnographic study that examines how hospital staff understands and manages patient safety risk refers to the written and tacit ways of providing care as the "formal and informal logic of risk" that enables staff to conduct "the practical everyday work of getting on with the job" (p. 367) [49]. I suggest that there is heuristic value in anthropomorphizing the hospital and in assigning to it agency as opposed to referring to contextual factors or hospital culture that are harder to define and discern in research. The advantage of identifying the hospital's discretionary power and its practical manifestations as agency allows us to recognize the hospital's intentionality to differentially treat marginalized and stigmatized patients (e.g., patients that can pose legal and resource risks for the institution and its providers by using street drugs in the hospital or by leaving AMA and becoming readmitted a short while later). Moreover, by assigned agency to the hospital, we can recognize how macro sociocultural factors (e.g., negative stereotypes associated with drug use) influence explicit hospital policies (e.g., prohibiting methadone maintenance treatment in the hospital or immediately calling security when a patient with SUD expresses a desire to leave the hospital) and implicit hospital practices (e.g., hospital administration not prioritizing the hiring of physicians specialized in addiction medicine or delaying placing a patient in a room because of staff concerns that the immediately available room is too close to the "narc" cabinet). The only way to elicit such tacit hospital features is through institutional ethnography.

Specifically, I suggest that institutional ethnography is an ideal method for identifying less obvious hospital features and tacit hospital processes and exploring how they influence patient-provider interactions but also are influenced by macro sociocultural forces (e.g., societal stigma assigned to HIV or psychiatric illness). The focus of this method on the texts institutions generate is especially useful in understanding AMA events [50, 51]. For instance, AMA signed forms or provider notes on AMA events routinely entered into patient electronic medical records are such texts, and they reflect institutional mandates and processes (e.g., what to do and what to write in the records when a patient expresses a desire to leave the hospital AMA). Such textual artifacts related to AMA events can reveal aspects of the workings of a hospital such as its professional hierarchy that emerges in how staff manages an AMA discharge. As mentioned earlier, our own content analysis of AMA notes written by different staff (e.g., nurses, residents, and attending physicians) demonstrated that nurses tended to call upon residents or attending physicians and residents called upon attending physicians to ask them to avert the AMA event or at least to cosign the AMA form and, thus, share the responsibility of the event with a colleague higher up in the hierarchy [36]. Although not articulated by providers as such, our analysis of the AMA notes revealed the hospital as an institution in the background of everything that providers did and recorded in relation to an AMA event. This implies that concern about institutional blame or at least institutional accountability informs provider habitus and behavior when patients challenge the normative hospital stay process by wanting to leave AMA.

Institutional texts can also reflect macro social policies and processes that extend beyond hospital walls [15, 16, 52]. For instance, the policy that excludes AMA discharges from the formula being used to calculate hospital penalties associated with 30-day readmissions combined with the lack of standards for classifying a discharge as AMA can undermine hospital incentives to devote extensive resources to avert such events. This policy suggests an implicit blaming of patients for the AMA discharge, a societal attitude that influences patient-provider interactions pertaining to an AMA event. Moreover, this implicit attitude can also emerge in the content and tone of the notes providers write following an AMA event. Societal attitudes toward patients who are discharged AMA can also be reflected in whether hospitals routinely write in the records whether the admitted patient has a history of AMA that often signals to providers a risk of a subsequent AMA event and can make them hypervigilant and suspicious when interacting with such a patient. Textual analysis of such routine entries in patient records enables institutional ethnographers to identify manifestations of a hospital's agency that shape provider habitus and, in turn, patient-provider interactions. As Sinding [14] suggested, institutional ethnography renders "visible how the work of people in a setting is coordinated textually, drawing on the knowledge various participants in a setting have on how to do things, and why things are done the way they are" (p. 1658). Therefore, combining textual analysis with the other ethnographic methods, that is, observations and in-depth interviews, we can identify hospital policies and tacit routines that set the context in which patient-provider interactions around an AMA event unfold. Being able to discern the hospital's agency will more accurately reveal how the institutional context shapes the patient-provider interactions that result in AMA discharges that amplify health disparities.

Conclusion and Next Steps

An AMA discharge is a complex phenomenon generated at the interface of the patient *habitus from the margins* and the provider *habitus, an amalgam of uncertainty and medical authority*. The patient-provider interactions shaped by their habitus are influenced by the *hospital's institutional agency* that reflects the large sociocultural context. The sociocultural context tolerates if not reproduces health disparities. Moreover, an AMA discharge indicates a rupture in the patient-provider interaction and a failure of the healthcare system to provide patient-centered care. Therefore, by studying AMA events, we can discern the mechanisms operating on the individual, interpersonal, institutional, and social levels that undermine the provision of patient-centered care and contribute to health disparities. AMA events provide the rare opportunity to understand how these four levels interact, and therefore, I consider them Mertonian strategic research events that illuminate how health inequities are produced, a fundamental and challenging public health and epidemiological question.

On an optimistic note, I want to remind the reader that an AMA discharge can generate the prospects for practice transformation to combat disparities. It can reveal to the patient and the provider each other's habitus and improve patient-provider understanding, enhance provider humility, and expose the institutional changes that will enable providers and systems to better care for the most vulnerable patients.

References

1. Glasgow JM, Vaughn-Sarrazin M, Kaboli PJ. Leaving against medical advice (AMA): risk of 30-day mortality and hospital readmission. J Gen Intern Med. 2010;25:926–9.
2. Ibrahim SA, Kwoh CK, Krishnan E. Factors associated with patients who leave acute-care hospitals against medical advice. Am J Public Health. 2007;97:2204–8.
3. Anis AH, Sun H, Guh DP, Palepu A, Schechter MT, O'Shaughnessy MV. Leaving hospital against medical advice among HIV-positive patients. Can Med Assoc J. 2002;167:633–7.
4. Baptist AP, Warrier I, Arora R, Ager J, Massanari RM. Hospitalized patients with asthma who leave against medical advice: characteristics, reasons, and outcomes. J Allergy Clin Immunol. 2007;119:924–9.
5. Alfandre DJ. "Im Going Home": discharges against medical advice. Mayo Clin Proc. 2009;84:255–60.

6. Franks P, Meldrum S, Fiscella K. Discharges against medical advice. J Gen Intern Med. 2006. https://doi.org/10.1111/j.1525-1497.2006.00505.x.
7. Kraut A, Fransoo R, Olafson K, Ramsey CD, Yogendran M, Garland A. A population-based analysis of leaving the hospital against medical advice: incidence and associated variables. BMC Health Serv Res. 2013. https://doi.org/10.1186/1472-6963-13-415.
8. Spooner KK, Salemi JL, Salihu HM, Zoorob RJ. Discharge against medical advice in the United States, 2002–2011. Mayo Clin Proc. 2017;92:525–35.
9. Tawk R, Freels S, Mullner R. Associations of mental, and medical illnesses with against medical advice discharges: the National Hospital Discharge Survey, 1988–2006. Admin Pol Ment Health. 2013;40:124–32.
10. Bourdieu P. Outline of a theory of practice. Cambridge, UK: Cambridge University Press; 1977.
11. Bourdieu P. The logic of practice. Stanford: Stanford University Press; 1990.
12. Lutfey Spencer K, Grace M. Social foundations of health care inequality and treatment bias. Ann Rev Sociol. 2016;42:101–20.
13. Freese J, Lutfey K. Fundamental causality: challenges of an animating concept for medical sociology. In: Handbook of the sociology of health, illness, and healing handbooks of sociology and social research. New York: Springer; 2011. p. 67–81.
14. Sinding C. Using institutional ethnography to understand the production of health care disparities. Qual Health Res. 20:1656–63.
15. Smith DE. Institutional ethnography: a sociology for people. Toronto: AltaMira Press; 2005.
16. van der Geest S, Finkler K. Hospital ethnography: introduction. Social Sci Med. 2004;59:1995–2001.
17. Merton RK. Three fragments from a sociologists notebooks: establishing the phenomenon, specified ignorance, and strategic research materials. Ann Rev Sociol. 1987;13:1–29.
18. Chan ACH, Palepu A, Guh DP, Sun H, Schechter MT, Oshaughnessy MV, Anis AH. HIV-positive injection drug users who leave the hospital against medical advice. JAIDS J Acquir Immune Defic Syndr. 2004;35:56–9.
19. Southern WN, Nahvi S, Arnsten JH. Increased risk of mortality and readmission among patients discharged against medical advice. Am J Med. 2012;125:594–602.
20. Crawford ND, White K, Rudolph AE, Jones KC, Benjamin EO, Fuller CM. The relationship between multiple forms of discrimination, neighborhood characteristics, and depression among illicit drug users in New York City. J Drug Issues. 2014;44:197–211.
21. Lekas H-M, Siegel K, Leider J. Felt and enacted stigma among HIV/HCV-coinfected adults. Qual Health Res. 2011;21:1205–19.
22. Pescosolido BA, Medina TR, Martin JK, Long JS. The "Backbone" of stigma: identifying the global core of public prejudice associated with mental illness. Am J Public Health. 2013;103:853–60.
23. Corrigan PW, Markowitz FE, Watson AC. Structural levels of mental illness stigma and discrimination. Schizophr Bull. 2004;30:481–91.
24. Hatzenbuehler ML, Phelan JC, Link BG. Stigma as a fundamental cause of population health inequalities. Am J Public Health. 2013;103:813–21.
25. Livingston JD, Boyd JE. Correlates and consequences of internalized stigma for people living with mental illness: a systematic review and meta-analysis. Soc Sci Med. 2010;71:2150–61.
26. Room R. Stigma, social inequality and alcohol and drug use. Drug Alcohol Rev. 2005;24:143–55.
27. Alfandre D, Yang J, Harwood K, Gordon P, Lekas H-M, Chang SJ, Yin MT. "Against Medical Advice" discharges among HIV-infected patients: health and health services outcomes. J Assoc Nurse AIDS Care. 2017;28:95–104.
28. Jeremiah J, O'Sullivan P, Stein MD. Who leaves against medical advice? J Gen Intern Med. 1995;10:403–5.

29. Haywood C, Lanzkron S, Hughes MT, Brown R, Massa M, Ratanawongsa N, Beach MC. A video-intervention to improve clinician attitudes toward patients with sickle cell disease: the results of a randomized experiment. J Gen Intern Med. 2010;26:518–23.
30. Haywood C, Lanzkron S, Ratanawongsa N, Bediako SM, Lattimer-Nelson L, Beach MC. Hospital self-discharge among adults with sickle-cell disease (SCD): associations with trust and interpersonal experiences with care. J Hosp Med. 2010;5:289–94.
31. Green P, Watts D, Poole S, Dhopesh V. Why patients sign out against medical advice (AMA): factors motivating patients to sign out AMA. Am J Drug Alcohol Abuse. 2004;30:489–93.
32. Onukwugha E, Saunders E, Mullins CD, Pradel FG, Zuckerman M, Weir MR. Reasons for discharges against medical advice: a qualitative study. BMJ Qual Saf Health Care. 2010;19:420–4.
33. Rentsch D, Luthy C, Perneger TV, Allaz A-F. Hospitalisation process seen by patients and health care professionals. Soc Sci Med. 2003;57:571–6.
34. Mcneil R, Small W, Wood E, Kerr T. Hospitals as a 'risk environment': an ethno-epidemiological study of voluntary and involuntary discharge from hospital against medical advice among people who inject drugs. Soc Sci Med. 2014;105:59–66.
35. Jerrard DA, Chasm RM. Patients leaving against medical advice (AMA) from the emergency department-disease prevalence and willingness to return. J Emerg Med. 2009;41:412–7.
36. Lekas H-M, Alfandre D, Gordon P, Harwood K, Yin MT. The role of patient-provider interactions: using an accounts framework to explain hospital discharges against medical advice. Soc Sci Med. 2016;156:106–13.
37. Alfandre D, Schumann JH. What is wrong with discharges against medical advice (and how to fix them). JAMA. 2013;310:2393.
38. Bartley MK. Against medical advice. J Trauma Nurs. 2014;21:314–8.
39. Berger JT. Discharge against medical advice: ethical considerations and professional obligations. J Hosp Med. 2008;3:403–8.
40. Devitt PJ, Devitt AC, Dewan M. An examination of whether discharging patients against medical advice protects physicians from malpractice charges. Psychiatr Serv. 2000;51:899–902.
41. Stern TW, Silverman BC, Smith FA, Stern TA. Prior discharges against medical advice and withdrawal of consent. Prim Care Companion CNS Disord. 2011. https://doi.org/10.4088/pcc.10f01047blu.
42. Levy F, Mareiniss DP, Iacovelli C. The importance of a proper against-medical-advice (AMA) discharge: how signing out AMA may create significant liability protection for providers. J Emerg Med. 2012;43:516–20.
43. Alfandre D. Reconsidering against medical advice discharges: embracing patient-centeredness to promote high quality care and a renewed research agenda. J Gen Intern Med. 2013;28:1657–62.
44. Schaefer GR, Matus H, Schumann JH, Sauter K, Vekhter B, Meltzer DO, Arora VM. Financial responsibility of hospitalized patients who left against medical advice: medical urban legend? J Gen Intern Med. 2012;27:825–30.
45. Windish DM, Ratanawongsa N. Providers' perceptions of relationships and professional roles when caring for patients who leave the hospital against medical advice. J Gen Intern Med. 2008;23:1698–707.
46. Berg KM, Arnsten JH, Sacajiu G, Karasz A. Providers' experiences treating chronic pain among opioid-dependent drug users. J Gen Intern Med. 2009;24:482–8.
47. Merrill JO, Rhodes LA, Deyo RA, Marlatt GA, Bradley KA. Mutual mistrust in the medical care of drug users. The keys to the "Narc" cabinet. J Gen Intern Med. 2002;17:327–33.
48. Ti L, Milloy M-J, Turje RB, Montaner J, Wood E, Kerr T. The impact of an HIV/AIDS adult integrated health program on leaving hospital against medical advice among HIV-positive people who use illicit drugs. J Public Health. 2016. https://doi.org/10.1093/pubmed/fdw057.
49. Dixon-Woods M, Suokas A, Pitchforth E, Tarrant C. An ethnographic study of classifying and accounting for risk at the sharp end of medical wards. Soc Sci Med. 2009;69:362–9.
50. Campbell ML. Institutional ethnography and experience as data. Qual Sociol. 1998;21:55–73.

51. Rankin J, Campbell M. Institutional ethnography (IE), nursing work and hospital reform: IE's cautionary analysis. Forum Qualitative Sozialforschung/Forum: Qual Soc Res. 2009;10(2). http://doi.org/10.17169/fqs-10.2.1258
52. Long D, Hunter C, Geest SVD. When the field is a ward or a clinic: hospital ethnography. Anthropol Med. 2008;15:71–8.

Chapter 6
Social Justice and the Ethics of Care: A Nursing Perspective

Jamie L. Shirley

Introduction

Healthcare systems are increasingly recognizing the importance of well-orchestrated transitions between care settings to promote quality outcomes. In this era of accountable care organizations and monitored hospital readmission rates, it is no longer possible to understand our responsibility for patients as ending at the door of the hospital. Multiple strategies are being explored to facilitate the coordination of care, and nurses are increasingly taking leadership roles in this work [1]. Both within the hospital and across long-term, home, and community health settings, nurses are positioned to collaborate in interprofessional teams to assist patients and their families to access the information and resources they need to make transitions successfully [2].

When patients are seeking early hospital discharge against the advice of their clinical team (or more commonly, are being discharged against medical advice [AMA]), nurses have a critical role in ensuring that care is being coordinated within the institution—that communication is effective, that appropriate resources are mobilized—and beyond to community settings—that referrals to needed services are made, and that patients have the means to actually access this care. Additionally, nurses can be instrumental in planning for the likely readmission of the patient in the future. Finally, nurses should consider how the design of their health system itself creates the conditions that precipitate AMA discharges and how policies and practices can be changed to enhance patient-centered care.

Thinking carefully about patients who seek AMA discharges illuminates the many contradictions within the healthcare system and, more specifically, the nursing role, which apply not only to these patients but to all our patients. These patient situations bring us face-to-face with our self-image as caring and trusted patient

J. L. Shirley (✉)
School of Nursing and Health Studies, University of Washington Bothell, Bothell, WA, USA
e-mail: jamiegs@uw.edu

© Springer International Publishing AG, part of Springer Nature 2018
D. Alfandre (ed.), *Against-Medical-Advice Discharges from the Hospital*,
https://doi.org/10.1007/978-3-319-75130-6_6

73

advocates. They call out our conflicted discursive language of personal responsibility and choice which is often in contradiction with our commitment to social justice. They bring our attention to our institutions' fiscal goals for efficient and timely discharges that also meet expectations for quality and safety.

Theoretical Context

Two theoretical threads inform nursing practice regarding patients who seek discharge against medical advice: social justice and the ethics of care. Both perspectives have deep historical roots in the nursing profession. Although both are largely congruent with the concept of patient-centered care, they also make visible some of its problematic aspects as will be discussed below.

Social Justice

Nursing traces its commitment to social justice to nineteenth- and twentieth-century reformers, such as Lavinia Dock and Lillian Wald, who understood the work of nursing to be inextricably linked to the obligation to address the social conditions that create health disparities [3]. This commitment is explicitly articulated in the ANA *Code of Ethics for Nurses* [4] and in AACN's *Essentials of Baccalaureate Education* [5]. These documents assert the responsibility of nurses to be leaders in promoting social conditions and health policies that ensure equitable access to health and healthcare.

Nurses are aware of the social inequities that shape the decisions and discharge options for patients. Patients who are discharged AMA are more likely to be those who are already socially marginalized—by income and class, by race and ethnicity, or by their status as substance users [6, 7]. These patients come into the hospital already at greater risk for poor health due to social disparities. Within the system, patients from these groups also report experiences of stigma and discrimination that make them less likely to trust their providers or engage in negotiated decision-making [8–10]. Upon discharge, their care options are likely to be limited by both availability and affordability. The perceived inability of nurses to address these social forces is often a source of considerable moral distress.

Ethics of Care

Nursing has long taken up the ethics of care as a moral foundation for its practice. Central to this model is the concept that relationships are not only an outcome, or a practical mechanism for achieving outcomes, but are the fundamental moral means by which we do our work [11]. Relationships are formed in interpersonal and social contexts and are central to human flourishing. One of the key elements of care is recognition—the identification of the moral agency of another (in this case the patient) and thus their right to make moral claims [12].

Aligned with this foundational conception of care is the understanding that personal identity is necessarily contingent [13]. That is, we can only understand our identity relationally—to the extent that we can make ourselves visible to another through the creation of sense-making narratives. When we create moral narratives together, these stories do not necessarily resolve disagreement, but they can help all parties to "acknowledge what commitments they are taking responsibility for and which understandings they refuse, foreclose, or silence" [14, p. 131].

This moral positioning is both congruent and at odds with the language of patient-centered care. On one hand, "patient-centered care" calls for exactly this kind of moral work. Patient-centered care accounts for patients' values, beliefs and commitments, their particular health needs, and their familial and social context. This kind of care requires recognition of and relational engagement with the moral agency of the patient. The hope is that by listening deeply and well to patients that we can mutually negotiate a plan of care that will lead to their improved health.

Unfortunately, this idea of patient-centered care can also slip into the language of autonomy, personal responsibility, and choice that can make social oppression and inequities less visible [15]. Choice is only a meaningful concept if the patient has access to a range of genuine options. The patient who works a job without sick leave or health insurance may not see staying in the hospital as a viable choice when weighed against the economic need to return to work. Similarly, a patient with substance abuse issues will find it difficult to take personal responsibility for her addiction recovery if there are no affordable rehabilitation programs available. In this context, nurses struggle with feelings of impotence, the feeling that the nurse, regardless of her disciplinary intentions or political actions, can have no immediate effect on the grand social problems faced by patients.

Nursing Role in AMA Discharges

If not effectively managed, the moral distress that nurses experience in these situations can be turned back onto the patients. The ready availability of the language of autonomy and responsibility exacerbates this tendency. Rather than maintaining a contextualized understanding of the patient's identity and situation, patients may instead be blamed for making irresponsible or unreasonable choices—thus allowing the nurse to abandon the professional obligation to remain relationally engaged. When this happens, the likelihood of achieving a positive outcome for the patient is diminished.

Over time, the nurse may also have her own sense of moral agency degraded [16]. Nurses are accustomed to being "the most trusted profession" [17]. When patients seemingly refuse the care we have to offer, when they reject our offers of engagement, it is all too easy to become punitive, to locate the problem in the patient, and to justify our dismissal of their needs. "Fine! We've tried our best to help you, but if you don't want our help…just go then!" While such a response may be momentarily satisfying, it ultimately harms the moral standing of both the patient and the nurse.

The task then for the nurse is to identify what can be done. Varcoe, Browne, and Cender advise understanding situations of structural inequity as practice problems and avoiding locating them exclusively in the patient (the difficult patient), the self (too inexperienced), or the institutional context (understaffed) [18]. If the ideal discharge is no longer an option, how can we make this a better discharge within the given constraints?

Understand Social Context

Understanding the context of the patient's desire for discharge has three levels. First, the nurse needs to explore the social and cultural context of the patient outside the hospital. Who forms the patient's support network? Are there people he is responsible for providing support to? What values and beliefs about health and healthcare does she bring? How is the patient affected by social disparities or oppression in the community? It is unlikely that the nurse can do anything to change these external conditions in this specific encounter, but knowing what they are can inform practice. Nurses need this knowledge to be able to share narratives with patients and their caregivers that will allow a common treatment plan to be negotiated [16].

Within the hospital, the hierarchies of power and other structural factors that affect the patient's experience also should be evaluated. We need to be alert to the possibility that the patient is not being unreasonable, but rather that she is responding to real experiences of structural racism or discrimination prevalent in healthcare settings [8]. Is the culture of the institution exacerbating the prior vulnerabilities of the patient? Are there barriers to meeting the patient's identified needs? Are there entrenched practices that are not based in evidence but are simply "how we do it here" that could be changed to accommodate this patient?

Those same hierarchies of power need to be evaluated for their constraints on the nurse's practice. Are there structural barriers to the robust interprofessional collaboration that these cases need? In recent years we have gotten better at rating patient acuity as a strategy to address staffing ratios, but these often fail to account for the psychosocial needs of patients. We need to acknowledge and accept that even a relatively stable patient can need more time. If the team's relationship with a patient is starting to decline, the sooner the nurse can make the commitment to put in the time to build and strengthen that relationship, the more likely there will be a positive outcome.

Commit to Creative Action

Patients in these situations need us to be creative and willing to alter our standard care patterns. The routinization of care is increasingly being advocated as a strategy to avoid errors, improve efficiency, and maintain high quality care. This approach, however, should not impede our ability to adapt that care to the specific needs of a patient. This is particularly true when the standard patterns of care create a marginalizing experience for a patient. "Equity is a goal that is never fully attained....but it is possible to promote in every moment, situation, and context" [18, p. 272]. What is one thing the nurse could do to make this situation better? It is difficult to know in advance what the turning point in a case will be—the particular intervention that will help the patient trust the system and agree to stay—or at least to stay long enough to arrange a safer, more controlled discharge.

Provide Consistency

If relationships are the heart of patient-centered care, then patients and nurses need the opportunity to build those relationships of trust through persistent engagement. We need staffing patterns that will accommodate this consistency. In the current system, most nurses are working 12 hour shifts, so patients rarely have the same nurse more than two days in a row, and few hospitals still have a robust system of primary nursing. For patients who are at risk for an AMA discharge, staffing should be managed to provide as much stability as possible. Our information management systems are increasingly effective at helping us communicate among the team, but sharing information well is not a substitute for building strong interpersonal bonds with patients.

Collaborate with Multiple Disciplines

Almost every case benefits from the work of a robust interdisciplinary team. In cases where a patient is contemplating an AMA discharge, they are particularly beneficial. Often these patients are angry at the primary team of doctors and nurses; they feel betrayed, lied to, or have come to see these clinicians as the source of their distress. Bringing in other providers who can build a bridge between the team and the patient is often helpful. This might be the behavioral health team, a social worker, or a chaplain. When available, a palliative care team or ethics consultant can sometimes fill this role. Of course, it is important to avoid splitting the team by the introduction of these additional participants—and many clinicians fear, particularly when ethics is included, that they will be told they have been doing it badly. Bringing in other disciplines can provide fresh perspectives on a case and break up the us/them dynamic that has often been created by the time an AMA discharge is being contemplated. The more interdisciplinarity is normalized, the less hierarchical the institution becomes. This flattening of power dynamics has benefits for not only the team but also the patient as communication becomes more honest, direct, and transparent.

Attend to Care Transitions

Care coordination is one of the "traditional strengths of the nursing profession" [19, p. 65]. Patients need their care to be coordinated both within the hospital and upon discharge. The issue of nursing consistency was addressed above, but there are many transitions of care within the hospital. From the patient's perspective, their care team can seem like a constantly mutating collection of staff. Medical teams rotate out and new ones come in; consultants appear once or twice and then disappear; nursing staff are present for long shifts but may not be consistent from day to day; social workers and chaplains are more likely to be consistent but are infrequent visitors. Patients need to know that all these staff members are communicating with each other and need to get consistent information about their plan of care. Nurses play a pivotal role in translating these staffing transitions to patients and ensuring that communication is effective so that important information is not lost.

Nurses can also be leaders in the effort to build meaningful relationships with the hospital's community partners. Discharge planning should not be an ad hoc process but should be guided by deep knowledge of external resources and an effort to effectively match the patient to the services that will best meet his needs. Outpatient and home-based providers can work with institutional partners to develop strategies to serve these infrequent, but not unexpected, patients.

Plan for the Next Admission

One of the most effective things nurses can do is to plan beyond this admission for the next one. A high percentage of patients who are discharged AMA return for a second admission, so we can anticipate that a patient who struggled to remain on the floor or who actually left early is likely to return. The temptation at the point of departure is to wash our hands of this patient and say good riddance. Odds are, however, that they will return because whatever it is that brought them to the hospital the first admission has not been resolved (or they wouldn't have left AMA!). This is the time to make a plan for the patient's care based on what helped build trust during this admission. Arranging a meeting of care providers to put a care plan in place for the patient's inevitable return to the hospital is time well spent. The care plan can alert the future providers to the patient's needs, preferences, and history so that the lessons learned on this admission are not lost.

Bringing interdisciplinary providers together to create a strategy for the next admission can change the outcome of a future admission. An example of this was a patient who needed a surgical intervention but providers were concerned about her ability to successfully recover because she had a history of leaving AMA several times in the past. The providers feared that she would try to leave again before she had completely healed from the surgery. To avoid this outcome, the nurses who had cared for her on prior admissions orchestrated a meeting with a range of providers to create a plan with a broad range of resources. To keep her engaged in the hospital setting and her recovery, the plan included reaching out to her clergy in the community, contacting the art therapist to visit her, and ordering more physical therapy visits than would routinely be scheduled. Additionally, her home care teaching was initiated even before the surgery, so she could be discharged as quickly as possible—with no delay for teaching self-care and no risk that she would leave before knowing how to be safe. This plan was effective for two reasons. First, it kept her engaged and distracted during the hospitalization which prevented her from having time to think about her desire to go home. It also demonstrated to the patient that we were committed to her successful recovery.

Engage in Healthcare System Design and Policy

One of the recommendations of the IOM's *Future of Nursing* report is for nurses to lead and diffuse collaborative improvement efforts [19]. Another recommendation encourages nurses to take an active role in leading change in the design of the healthcare system. Patients who seek early discharge raise multiple questions for system change. The obvious quality improvement project is to seek strategies that help these patients complete their recommended hospital stay. However, the healthcare system as a whole potentially has more to learn from the opposite project. The desire for early discharge by patients is actually in alignment with the fiscal goals of the hospital. More and more we are seeking to discharge patients who do not need to be in the hospital and to provide their care in less restrictive, less risky, and less expensive environments. Can our efforts to facilitate safe discharges for this population help us to reimagine meaningful discharge options?

Because these patients represent only 1–2% of all hospitalizations, they are a difficult population to study. Many are lost to follow-up, and our impressions of their trajectory are anecdotal and potentially misleading. However, with the assistance of electronic medical records, nurses can track these patients over time to confirm or refute those impressions and develop care coordination interventions that facilitate improved outcomes.

Additionally, research on this population may help make visible the antecedents of their requests for early discharge. How do our current practices create the environment for these patients to feel disenfranchised and alienated by the healthcare system? Again, although these patients are a small fraction of the total patient population, they are acting out distress that is reported by a much broader population of patients.

Conclusion

Historically, we have spent time and effort developing interventions that we hope will change our patients and make them more amenable to our recommendations for care. Patients come to us for a brief time with complex narratives. There is so much we will not know about them—their history, their current context, and the impact on their future of their current choices. We can approach them with humility and curiosity—asking questions and seeking to build negotiated relationships. But ultimately, we would likely be better served by focusing on changing our own practice and institutions to make them more just and more responsive. There is much more we can do to create unobstructed pathways for them between illness and health and between home, hospital, and community.

References

1. Naylor MD. Advancing high value transitional care: the central role of nursing and its leadership. Nurs Adm Q. 2012;36(2):115–26. https://doi.org/10.1097/NAQ.0b013e31824a040b.
2. Cipriano P. The imperative for patient, family, and population-centered interprofessional approaches to care coordination and transitional care: a policy brief by the American Academy of Nursing's Care Coordination Task Force. Nurs Outlook. 2012;60(5):330–3.
3. Bekemeier B, Butterfield P. Unreconciled inconsistencies: a critical review of the concept of social justice in 3 national nursing documents. ANS Adv Nurs Sci. 2005;28(2):152–62.
4. American Nurses Association (ANA). Code of ethics for nurses. Washington, DC: American Nurses Association; 2015.
5. American Association of Colleges of Nursing (AACN). The essentials of baccalaureate education for professional nursing practice. Washington, DC: AACN; 2008.
6. Aliyu ZY. Discharge against medical advice: sociodemographic, clinical and financial perspectives. Int J Clin Pract. 2002;56(5):325–7.
7. Alfandre DJ. "I'm going home": discharges against medical advice. Mayo Clin Proc. 2009;84(3):255–60. https://doi.org/10.1016/S0025-6196(11)61143-9.
8. Institute of Medicine (IOM). Unequal treatment: confronting racial and ethnic disparities in health care. Washington, DC: National Academies Press; 2002.
9. van Ryn M, Burke J. The effect of patient race and socio-economic status on physicians' perceptions of patients. Soc Sci Med. 2000;50(6):813–28.
10. van Boekel LC, Brouwers EP, van Weeghel J, Garretsen HF. Stigma among health professionals towards patients with substance use disorders and its consequences for healthcare delivery: systematic review. Drug Alcohol Depend. 2013;131(1–2):23–35. https://doi.org/10.1016/j.drugalcdep.2013.02.018.
11. Tronto JC. Moral boundaries: a political argument for an ethic of care. New York: Routledge; 1993.
12. Walker M. How relationships heal. In: Walker M, Rosen WB, editors. How connections heal: stories from relational-cultural therapy. New York: Guildford Press; 2004.
13. Lindemann NH. Damaged identities, narrative repair. Ithaca: Cornell University; 2001.
14. Walker MU. Moral contexts. Lanham: Rowen & Littlefield; 2003.
15. Doane GH. Cultivating relational consciousness in social justice practice. In: Kagan PN, Smith MC, Chinn PL, editors. Philosophies and practices of emancipatory nursing: social justice as praxis. New York: Routledge; 2014. p. 241–50.

16. Liaschenko J. Making a bridge: the moral work with patients we do not like. J Palliat Care. 1994;10(3):83–9.
17. Gallup Poll. Americans rate nurses highest on honesty, ethical standards. 2014. http://news.gallup.com/poll/180260/americans-rate-nurses-highest-honesty-ethical-standards.aspx. Accessed 18 Jul 2017.
18. Varcoe C, Browne AJ, Cender LM. Promoting social justice and equity by practicing nursing to address structural inequities and structural violence. In: Kagan PN, Smith MC, Chinn PL, editors. Philosophies and practices of emancipatory nursing: social justice as praxis. New York: Routledge; 2014. p. 266–84.
19. Institute of Medicine (IOM). The future of nursing: leading change, advancing health. Washington, DC: National Academies Press; 2010.

Part II
Preventing and Managing Against Medical Advice Discharges Across the Spectrum of Care

Chapter 7
Bedside Management of Discharges Against Medical Advice

Holly Fleming, David S. Olson Jr., David Alfandre, and Cynthia Geppert

Physicians and other healthcare professionals have long struggled with discharges against medical advice (AMA), or when patients leave the hospital prior to a specified clinical end point over the recommendation of the physician. Recognition of the stress and anxiety associated with AMA discharge is described as early as the 1920s in the literature related to pulmonary tuberculosis patients who were leaving the tuberculosis sanitoria before completion of treatment. A psychiatric paper published in 1962 describes a clinician's struggle:

> Discharge against medical advice is a disruptive crisis on a psychiatric ward. The patient, his family, his fellow-patients, and the staff are often disappointed, frustrated and angry. If the discharge occurs early in the course of hospitalization, the painful sacrifices that have been made to bring about hospitalization seem to have been in vain. If it occurs later, many of the participants feel as if the maximum therapeutic benefits have not been derived. Such crisis often result in one or another segment of the staff being blamed for the undesirable outcome. [1]

The views expressed in this article are those of the authors and do not necessarily reflect the position or policy of the U.S. Department of Veterans Affairs, the US Government, or the VA National Center for Ethics in Health Care.

H. Fleming (✉)
Hospital Medicine, Raymond G. Murphy VA Medical Center, Albuquerque, NM, USA

University of New Mexico, Albuquerque, NM, USA
e-mail: Holly.fleming@va.gov

D. S. Olson Jr.
Department of Internal Medicine, Raymond G. Murphy VA Medical Center,
Albuquerque, NM, USA

D. Alfandre
VHA National Center for Ethics in Health Care, Department of Veterans Affairs,
NYU School of Medicine, New York, NY, USA

C. Geppert
New Mexico Veterans Affairs Health Care System, Department of Psychiatry
and Director of Ethics Education, Albuquerque, NM, USA

© Springer International Publishing AG, part of Springer Nature 2018
D. Alfandre (ed.), *Against-Medical-Advice Discharges from the Hospital*,
https://doi.org/10.1007/978-3-319-75130-6_7

85

There has been considerable research into the profile of the patient most likely to leave AMA as both the basis for developing interventions like the ones described in this chapter and to minimize the negative impact of the phenomenon. Demographic factors associated with AMA discharge were described in a *New England Journal of Medicine* article published in 1979, where the author identifies the "role of addiction" and "the finding of disproportionately high numbers of poor, single and black patients" as associated with AMA discharge [2]. This author recognized that "Early treatment of addiction, special attention to establishing relations with patients who tend toward alienation because of socioeconomic, ethnic or personality factors and early detection of brain syndromes and psychoses might be helpful measures in the prevention of discharge against advice" [2].

The ensuing decades have confirmed many of these same risk factors and correlates associated with AMA discharges. For example, in recent literature, risk factors for AMA discharge have been identified as previous AMA discharge, male sex, younger age, substance use disorders, mental health diagnosis, Medicaid or no insurance, and lower socioeconomic status [3–6]. Previous studies have consistently found that the most common reasons patients leave AMA are related to substance use disorders, financial or personal obligations, hospital fatigue, communication issues, perceived delays in care, and/or poor quality of care [5–8].

For several reasons, AMA discharge has received increased attention in the clinical and quality improvement literature over the last decade. The first is the association of AMA discharge with increased morbidity and mortality [3, 9–11]. Second, readmission rates for this high-risk cohort of patients are from two to seven times higher than patients discharged with medical approval, resulting in higher costs and use of more hospital resources [3, 4, 6, 9–11]. With an estimated 500,000 AMA discharges from hospitals each year, this places a strain on an already under-resourced healthcare system [12]. Finally, there are trends suggesting that the rates of AMA discharge are increasing, highlighting the need for more efforts directed toward improving patient safety and transitions of care for this high-risk patient population [13].

In this chapter, we first analyze some of the common barriers and misconceptions that may lead providers to pursue an AMA discharge. We then discuss the available evidence-based best practices and associated cognitive and behavioral strategies for responding to patients who request to leave the hospital AMA. Lastly, we outline how to apply these strategies to clinical practice.

Review of Literature

Historically, AMA discharges have been viewed by institutions as risk management events where, frequently, both patients and providers feel blamed for any undesirable outcomes. This perspective can often result in an adversarial relationship between the patient and treatment team from which no one benefits. Recent literature has identified and described numerous best practice approaches for an AMA discharge. In 2009, as part of a review of the topic, Alfandre outlined several core concepts or strategies for optimizing an AMA discharge [6]. These strategies included the following:

1. Addressing substance abuse
2. Recognizing psychological factors
3. Motivational interviewing
4. Informed consent
5. Arranging appropriate follow-up care

To our knowledge, this list of strategies was the first set of informal "guidelines" for managing AMA discharges. This guidance provided a dramatic conceptual change in the understanding of AMA discharge by emphasizing a patient-centered approach for discharge of this high-risk group of patients. This approach promoted shared decision-making (SDM) in discharge planning as a tool to manage disagreements between patients and providers. In SDM, clinicians are advised to "identify a specific clinical problem, gauge patients' preferences for involvement in the decision-making process, elicit patients' values and preferences for care, and then identify a range of medically appropriate options for management of that clinical problem" [14]. As an approach to managing AMA discharges, SDM allows for better understanding of the often unrecognized socioeconomic and emotional factors that may drive a patient's decision to leave.

The goal of these strategies is to address patient needs and mitigate provider and institutional concerns. Even when these strategies do not result in more patients remaining in the hospital to complete treatment, which is the primary objective, they can be used to help patients leave the hospital with safer discharge plans. This safer transition of care is a secondary objective and, perhaps in the long term, a more important one.

A crucial aspect of this conceptualization of AMA discharge is recognition of the central role that substance use disorders play in many clinical and ethical conflicts between patients and medical teams. Additionally, studies have identified that patients with substance use disorders are often readmitted multiple times and are, therefore, very high utilizers of limited healthcare resources [3, 4, 6, 9–11]. Inadequate treatment of pain, particularly in patients with a history of addiction who have developed a tolerance to opioid medication or symptoms of withdrawal, is a common reason that patients report leaving AMA [5]. Lack of provider education related to management of addiction and pain may create standoffs or stalemates in which practitioners perceiving patients as making unreasonable demands for controlled substances, react with angry rebuffs leading to the breakdown of the patient-physician relationship. To avoid such ruptures in the treatment relationship, it is imperative to approach these patients with empathy and with a nonjudgmental attitude. Consultation early in the admission, with psychiatry and/or with pain management/addiction specialists, should be obtained to optimize care for these patients.

Recognizing specific psychological factors contributing to the emotional distress patients experience when they are sick and hospitalized is another important strategy in the effort to prevent an AMA discharge. The request or threat to leave AMA has been described as a way for patients to demonstrate their feelings of anger, anxiety, or depression [6]. Failure to recognize and address psychological disturbances can lead to a negative patient-provider relationship. Motivational interviewing is a technique in which the provider uses "nonjudgmental, empathetic questioning to uncover the unspoken motivations behind patient's particular behaviors" [6]. Understanding patient motivation allows the provider to focus on interventions that may lead to the negotiation of a more appropriate discharge plan.

For example, a patient may exhibit far more concern about leaving the hospital to pay the rent on time than the need to stay in the hospital to complete treatment for community-acquired pneumonia. In this scenario, recognizing that the patient has good reason to leave the hospital, the provider can request that social work assist the patient to pay his rent or to ensure that allowances are made. This strategy enables the provider to focus on clinical concerns. Demonstrating respect for the patients' priorities and the attempt to balance these with the clinical need to remain in the hospital may result in strengthening the patient-provider relationship. Often, this is enough to convince the patient to remain in the hospital, even if immediate arrangements cannot be made. Together, these two interventions may convey to the patient that the provider cares about him as a person and thereby, prevent the AMA discharge. As an example of SDM, this interaction demonstrates how to take patient preferences into consideration and to empathize with the patient's perspective when identifying and discussing treatment options.

When negotiating with a patient about leaving the hospital AMA, a clinically sound informed consent is essential both legally and ethically. Informed consent ensures that patients are informed about their care so that they can make voluntary decisions in accordance with their own values and interests. This includes an understanding of the indication for the treatment, its risks and benefits, as well as the risks and benefits of the alternatives. As part of informed consent, patients have the right to accept or decline recommended treatments, even life-sustaining treatments. Informed consent or refusal requires three core elements: (1) The provider discloses adequate information delivered in a way the patient can comprehend. (2) The patient has intact decision-making capacity. (3) The patient is able to make a voluntary choice [15]. We will briefly examine each element as it relates to AMA discharges. The components of decisional capacity and requirements for an informed consent discussion are summarized below [15].

Decisional Capacity Assessment

The patient must be able to:

- Communicate preferences
- Comprehend the gravity of the situation and decisions
- Reason through and manipulate information
- Make choices reflecting personal values, free of coercion

Elements of an Informed Consent Discussion

- A clear diagnosis and prognosis is explained to the patient.
- An explanation of the nature of the intervention.
- An explanation of the risks of the intervention.
- An explanation of the benefits of the intervention.
- Alternatives to the intervention and their risks and benefits, including no intervention.

Performing and documenting a thorough informed consent discussion is a critical component of managing an AMA discharge and has been shown to be more legally protective than the use of a generic AMA form [16, 17]. However, there is variation in provider comfort level and education when obtaining informed consent because of difficulty in assessing decisional capacity. Assessment of decisional capacity can be the most challenging aspect of conducting an informed consent discussion, especially for nonpsychiatric physicians. Although physicians often raise decisional capacity concerns when patients fail to agree with their medical recommendations, they are much less likely to do so when the patient agrees with their recommendation. The goal in a capacity assessment is to evaluate the *process* through which a patient makes a decision far more than the *content* of the decision. Therefore, a capacity assessment may be indicated in a patient with known major neurocognitive impairment, even if they agree with the physician's recommendation [18]. When patients do not follow provider recommendations, providers often make the assumption that they do not "care about their health," which can be understandably frustrating for providers. It may help providers to realize that, more commonly, patients are choosing a competing value, such as ensuring a companion animal is cared for or meeting a family obligation. These obligations are often more immediate and significant to the patient than medical considerations.

Patients have the right to make choices that appear to providers as "irrational", when those choices make sense in the context of their life history and values. The concept of informed refusal requires the provider to discuss the same information as when obtaining informed consent. Providers can utilize the concept of the "Sliding Scale of Informed Consent" to", assist them with assessing patient capacity to make different types of medical decisions [15]. This concept suggests that there should be a higher threshold of certainty of decisional capacity as the risk of an intervention increases or the benefits decrease. Therefore, lower-risk procedures or clinical scenarios require less demanding standards of decisional capacity (Fig. 7.1).

For example, high-risk prostate surgery for a slow-growing and potentially nonlethal cancer in an 82-year-old patient who is more likely to die of his advanced congestive heart failure is an intervention that is very high-risk with disputed benefits. There is expert clinical judgment that may support a decision to forgo this procedure that has many associated complications in an effort to address a cancer that may not shorten life expectancy. In this case, the bar for assessing the patient's decisional capacity is set very high. A provider must be certain that a patient understands the morbidity associated with the procedure, such as incontinence and

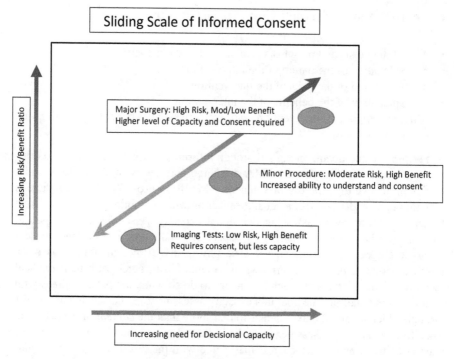

Fig. 7.1 Sliding scale of informed consent. This graphic demonstrates the concept that as the risk of an intervention increases relative to the benefits, the threshold for ensuring decisional capacity increases

erectile dysfunction. In this scenario, both informed consent and refusal require complex decision-making, and the capacity assessment would focus on the higher-order capacities of reasoning and appreciation. Additionally, when a patient refuses a very low-risk/high-benefit procedure such as a potentially lifesaving appendectomy for acute appendicitis, the bar for assessing the patient's decisional capacity is also set very high, and the provider must be quite certain that the patient is making a rational and voluntary refusal. To the contrary, an elderly woman who agrees to treatment for a urinary tract infection may require only lower-order capacities such as understanding the diagnosis and treatment and the ability to communicate a choice that she would like to be treated. When there is doubt or concern about decisional capacity, the provider can seek guidance from mental healthcare professionals with expertise in capacity assessment. For a patient to be discharged AMA, they must have decisional capacity and be able to participate in an informed consent discussion about declining further inpatient treatment. Strategies for managing patients who are threatening to elope from a facility and who lack decisional capacity are beyond the scope of this chapter.

Lastly, informed consent requires that the patient not only have adequate decisional capacity but also the ability to make voluntary choices without excessive internal or external coercion. Withholding information, providing misinformation, or threatening patients that they will no longer receive care or will be subject to excessive charges unless they remain hospitalized, undermines a patient's ability to make choices free of coercion and thus, reduces the quality of the informed consent.

Among the most common of such threats compromising voluntarism is the misperception that insurance companies will not reimburse for a hospitalization when a patient is discharged AMA. Two studies have addressed this concern. In 2008, Wigder reviewed 104 consecutive cases of patients with insurance leaving AMA from a suburban level I trauma center emergency department. All 104 emergency department visits where the patient was discharged AMA were fully reimbursed by every insurance company [19]. The largest retrospective cohort study to date, looking at provider perceptions and insurance reimbursement in relation to AMA discharge, was conducted at the University of Chicago [20]. In this study, approximately 526 (1%) of 46,319 patients admitted during the study period were discharged AMA. The number of patients discharged AMA who had insurance was 453 (86%). Of these, there were only 18 (4%) cases where insurance companies did not reimburse for services. Common reasons for payment denial included delayed submission of the bill, confusion about patient identity, and extended utilization review. There were no instances in which an insurance company denied payment because the patient left AMA [20]. In this same study, attending physicians and residents were surveyed and asked to respond to the statement "when a patient leaves the hospital against medical advice, insurance companies do not pay for the patient's hospitalization." Sixty-eight percent of residents and 44% of attending physicians "agreed" or "strongly agreed" with this statement. Those who believed that insurance would not pay for an AMA hospitalization reported that they would inform patients that they might be held financially responsible for the hospitalization so that the patient would "reconsider staying in the hospital" [20]. These studies support that insurance companies do in fact, most commonly, reimburse for AMA discharges. Nevertheless, this myth is very strongly associated with AMA discharge. How frequently providers use this threat to coerce patients to remain hospitalized is unknown.

The practice of arranging post-acute care for patients discharged AMA is another controversial topic. In clinical practice, a common misperception is that provider responsibility ends when a patient is discharged AMA. Furthermore, providers often believe that liability may actually increase if they are involved in facilitating the care transition. Bioethicists and many risk managers now support that AMA discharge should be treated like other care transitions in which the goal is to optimize patient safety during the transfer of care to the outpatient setting [21–23].

Quill argues that non-abandonment is one of a physician's central ethical obligations. He defines this concept as the "longitudinal commitment both to care about patients and to jointly seek solutions to problems with patients throughout their illness" [22]. Quill argues that the minimum requirement of this obligation is to ensure some form of continuity for the patient at discharge, but he also recognizes that the depth and nature of this commitment may vary for individual physicians and patients. Although Quill advocates for the concept of non-abandonment, he acknowledges that physicians should not violate their own values in taking care of the patient. To avoid such conflicts, he recommends that healthcare systems develop policies that "reinforce rather than undermine physicians' willingness to engage with patients when their problems seem insoluble, or in situations in which the problems are not clearly resolved through current ethical thinking and consultation" [22].

Other bioethicists support the concept of arranging post-acute care for AMA discharge as a professional obligation and point out that there is little evidence to support the concern that providing patients with aftercare resources exposes physicians or institutions to greater legal liability [21]. In fact, providers and institutions often fail to appreciate the potential liability associated with declining to provide aftercare that results in an adverse outcome. Berger argues that patients also have an obligation to use healthcare resources responsibly and to honor their commitments [21].

The advent of hospital medicine as a specialty resulted in significant improvement in efficiency of providing inpatient care. However, this model of providing care increased the number of patient "hand-offs" compared to the traditional model where a primary care provider would care for the same patient across the continuum of outpatient and inpatient settings. This healthcare model inherently limits the ability for physicians to maintain longitudinal relationships with patients. Regardless of this challenge, it does not negate that at minimum, every attempt should be made to optimize the transition of care back to the outpatient setting.

As part of this ambivalence about offering patients who leave AMA post-acute care, clinicians are often conflicted over whether to provide discharge medications. Some authors advocate that when good faith attempts to convince a patient to stay are exhausted, "the professional responsibility shifts to a sincere and meticulous effort to mitigate harm by providing the best possible alternative plan of care that the patient will accept" [23]. Physicians may decline to offer an alternative care plan because of concern over appearing to endorse substandard care [23] and then being held responsible legally and/or institutionally for any adverse outcome. However, such reasoning fails to consider the potential accountability of an untoward outcome that occurs precisely because of the providers' refusal to offer care.

Even suboptimal care may be superior to no care, which can be harmful to the patient and thus, breaches a physician's core ethical commitment. For example, a patient may refuse to stay in the hospital to complete a course of intravenous antibiotics but would consider taking an oral antibiotic with outpatient appointments for ongoing monitoring of treatment response. This treatment may not be the recommended standard, but if it is still within acceptable medical standards, then it is arguable that it may be better than no care. Protection from liability in this scenario again, rests in performance of a thorough informed consent discussion coupled with good documentation.

Translation into Clinical Practice

The current SDM literature supports strategies to optimize AMA discharges that share the common themes of patient needs assessment, decisional capacity assessment, documentation of informed consent discussions, and maximization of the transition of care back to the outpatient setting [6, 21–24]. Clark et al. (Table 7.1)

Table 7.1 A practical approach: AIMED

Assess
Severity of illness/urgency of treatment
Decision-making capacity (treat underlying cause if impaired)
Degree of risk to patient's health and welfare
Investigate
Patient's reason for leaving
Comfort (symptom management)
Communication regarding care plan
Withdrawal syndromes
Pressing responsibilities like child, elder, or pet care issue
Allies such as primary care provider or family member
Mitigate
Offer maximal necessary treatment acceptable to patient
Provide prescriptions for medications as indicated
Provide optimal follow-up plan and discharge instructions
Explain
Original treatment plan risks and benefits
Specific dangers of failing to follow proposed plan
Discharge instructions including reasons to return
That the patient is welcome to return at any time
Document
Medical screening exam
Decision-making capacity assessment
Discussion of initial treatment offered
Discussion of patient refusal and reasoning
Efforts to negotiate and recruit family/friends
Alternative plan with risks and benefits
Discharge instructions including when to return
Efforts to locate if no discharge conversation occurred

Reprinted from Clark et al. [23]. With permission from John Wiley and Sons

expanded on the strategies for optimizing an AMA discharge and developed an approach using the mnemonic AIMED that offered a concise and systematic method to meet the professional, legal, and ethical obligations that arise when patients decline medical care and request AMA discharge [23].

This mnemonic describing the steps that should be taken when a patient requests AMA discharge expands on the above bioethics strategies introduced in 2009 and emphasizes the importance of documentation. The authors specifically state that "the overriding goal of these responsibilities is to reduce the numbers of patients who ultimately leave before their medical care is complete and to reduce poor outcomes, patient morbidity, and dissatisfaction on the part of patients and providers" [23].

Behavioral and Cognitive Strategies

We will now outline a series of behavioral and cognitive strategies providers can utilize to manage patients who request to be discharged AMA. The behavioral strategies entail that clinicians change their actions, while the cognitive strategies entail clinicians to change their thinking. Both strategies are intended to empower the clinician to better manage AMA discharges but can also be challenging for clinicians to implement. These strategies seek to help clinicians focus on what they are doing at the bedside to work more productively with patients to promote better health outcomes.

Behavioral Strategies

1. *Involve other sources of support for the patient.*

If there is disagreement over the treatment plan and the clinician is working to persuade the patient to remain hospitalized, the clinician should involve with the patient's permission, the patient's family, friends, and others who the patient trusts. These individuals can be extraordinarily helpful allies in working productively with the patient to make decisions that promote the patient's health. This potential source of support is useful irrespective of whether the patient chooses to remain hospitalized or to leave with appropriate aftercare. Among these allies is the patient's primary care physician and/or other physicians with whom the patient has a strong and trusting relationship. These allies can sometimes be more effective than the healthcare team in convincing the patient that his choice to leave may not promote his overall goals or health outcomes.

2. *Maximize the amount of decisions the patient can control.*

Patients may choose to leave the hospital because they are no longer comfortable and willing to engage in inpatient treatment. The discomfort, indignities, and frustrations of inpatient hospitalization can leave a patient so exasperated, that they are willing to risk their health to promote their comfort. In this scenario, the patient perceives that they are actually making a positive choice for their well-being. Saying no to inpatient treatment may be the most powerful and effective way for a patient to assert control over their environment in the hospital. In recognizing this, clinicians can work to first address the patient's primary concern, whether it be about the physical environment, medication schedules or some other detail of the hospital routine. The team can also work to identify other areas that promote the patient's control over their environment in the hospital but do not present a similar risk to their health. Perhaps the patient wants to leave the unit to take a walk around the ward or the grounds? Perhaps the patient wants his medication dosed less frequently or fewer awakenings in the night so he can sleep better? Clinicians should be motivated to identify such areas where the patient can be made much more comfortable simply by encouraging the patient's involvement in the care plan.

3. *Empathize, do not argue.*

When patients first notify the healthcare staff that they are going to leave the hospital against a provider's recommendation, they are often already frustrated and sometimes angry about their hospital care. The most effective response in this situation is to empathize with the patient's position. Patients, more than anything, wish to be heard. Choosing to argue, no matter how well intentioned or even correct the provider may be, is not likely to convince the patient to stay and may strengthen the patient's resolve to leave. The clinician's goal is to align the healthcare team with the patient, and the most expedient way to do so is to remain open to the patient's concerns. Empathy can reduce the patient's sense of alienation and fear in hopes that they are less likely to fight with the healthcare team as a means of defending their interests. Empathy allows the clinician to see situations from the patient's perspective and work together to resolve the issues that led to the conflict. This process requires that the clinician redirect back to the patient's concerns and away from issues extraneous to the problem, even if the provider is technically correct about the hospital protocol or the delivery of a treatment.

4. *Rely on trusted legal advice about AMA discharges*

There is limited empirical data regarding clinician's overall knowledge, attitudes, and practices about AMA discharges. However, what is known from surveys is that many clinicians continue to believe that AMA discharges can confer protection from legal liability and thus, justify their use. It is possible that a heightened concern about liability affects clinician's motivation and ability to resolve the patient's concerns at the bedside. Although there are strong ethical rationales for avoiding the AMA discharge designation, many clinicians will not be persuaded until they have assurances that doing so will not expose them or their hospital to legal liability. For this reason, clinicians at their home institution should work closely with their hospital counsel and risk management to obtain specific and authoritative advice about the legal concerns in managing AMA discharges. This will help to assuage the legal concerns of burdened providers confronting challenging situations. If clinicians are less concerned about the legal issues in the patient care, they can more easily focus their attention on the comprehensive care of the patient which is, after all, what they are trained to do.

Cognitive Strategies

Many clinicians adhere to a patient-provider relationship model in which it is the clinician's task to provide patients with information and advice about how to promote their health, and it is the patient's job to follow that advice. In this model, if the patient chooses not to follow the clinician's recommendations, then the clinician has no further obligation to the patient. The cognitive strategies we propose challenge that line of reasoning. Because they offer a more productive way to interact with patients and to improve the quality of the patient-provider relationship, these cognitive strategies can improve both patient care and clinician well-being.

Part of why AMA discharges are so frustrating to clinicians is the feeling that it prevents them from accomplishing their task. This has been described in the social science literature as "role hindrance" [25]. There are socialized roles within society and medical practice that patients and providers are generally expected to fulfill. These positions and roles are socialized in that they are powerfully felt and enacted, even if not necessarily consciously recognized or articulated. When either party deviates from these roles, there is some form of distress. In this construct, it is the patient's role to dutifully follow a doctor's advice, and it is the doctor's role to help patients get well. Applying this construct to AMA discharges can help illuminate what about them causes distress and how best to address it.

The clinician's role, reinforced through the socialization of medicine, leads them to internalize this strong desire for patients to get better. Some clinicians, who are thwarted in this role, may experience this "role hindrance" and become overly frustrated with themselves and/or the patient. If role hindrance occurs frequently and consistently enough, it may contribute to professional burnout. These cognitive strategies are an attempt to improve patient outcomes, primarily by improving a clinician's ability to recognize the sources and nature of this distress and, therefore, be better equipped to constructively negotiate these challenging encounters.

1. *Conflict as opportunity*:

Although disagreements with patients can be challenging for some clinicians to address and manage, they are an inevitable part of patient care. Disagreements can derive from the patient's or clinician's behavior, patient expectations, or a patient's choice about treatment options. Factors outside of the control of either party, such as delays in referrals, can also lead to conflict. Lack of alignment between what the clinician recommends and what the patient wants, requests, or perceives is the hallmark of an AMA discharge. A patient typically requests AMA discharge when they are dissatisfied with a treatment plan that they believe is no longer is in accordance with or even contravening their values and interests. Regardless of the patient's reason for being dissatisfied, perhaps something as simple as unsavory meals, if the clinician approaches this conflict not as a reason to fight but as an opportunity to better engage with the patient, it may be easier to align with the patient and the overall goals of treatment. A request to leave AMA is often viewed as adversarial, but it can also be seen as an opportunity to connect with the patient. In requesting to leave AMA, a patient is attempting to articulate needs, wishes, and preferences for care. This attempt at connection should be welcomed, not rebuffed, ignored, or even ridiculed. The request to leave may simply be the beginning of a conversation about how best to meet the patient's needs, whatever they may be.

2. *Understanding and accepting patients with substance use disorders*

Consistently over time, the largest cohort of AMA discharges is among patients with a history of a substance use disorder. This population is heavily stigmatized for their illness, both in society and in the medical profession. Caring for this population may test a clinician's professionalism more than any other medical or psychiatric illness. Particularly challenging for clinicians is difficulty with the concept of "cure" in this population and the lower rates of treatment compliance and maintenance among these patients. Additionally, there still exists widespread belief, both within and outside of the medical community, that those struggling with addiction have a moral failing worthy of judgment rather than having a treatable medical illness. For these reasons, clinicians may find themselves with less understanding and acceptance of substance users and accordingly less motivation to help them manage their illnesses or persuade them to remain in the hospital.

Cultivating understanding and acceptance of patients with substance use disorders begins with the clinician's mindful admission of any bias toward this population. Recognizing one's biases makes it easier to counteract them. It is easier to feel empathy toward a person if one knows their background and history. Seeing patients as suffering individuals with unique backgrounds, families, and often tragic life stories, rather than simply a conglomeration of difficult to treat symptoms, facilitates better relationships and less provider helplessness and rejection. Finally, understanding helps clinicians accept the patient's experience living with and managing a substance use disorder. Understanding may help the provider feel less personal responsibility when the patient is unable or unwilling to remain hospitalized or continue treatment for their substance use disorder.

3. *Choice about discharge designation*

Although a patient with decision-making capacity has the authority to leave the hospital prior to a clinically specified end point, the decision to formally designate the discharge as AMA is at the discretion of the healthcare professional. The clinician's ethical and legal obligation to the patient is to ensure the patient is making an informed choice about declining inpatient treatment and to document it appropriately in the medical record. This may include a recommendation to remain hospitalized until a safer or more appropriate time as determined by the provider. Because designation of a discharge as AMA has not been demonstrated to improve patient care and there are increasingly recognized risks of reducing access and stigmatization associated with its use, some have advocated that it is ethically problematic to use the designation at all. The fact that there are no clear standards or definitions for what constitutes an AMA discharge further complicates the decision and may lead to a reduction in healthcare quality secondary to the clinical variability in the use of the term. Healthcare professionals should consider the benefits and burdens associated with the designation as it applies to the patients under their care, and choose whether or not the AMA discharge designation promotes the patient's best interest.

Case Vignettes

We now describe a series of case vignettes that illustrate how to apply the concepts introduced in this chapter, particularly the behavioral and cognitive strategies just reviewed.

Case 1

Mr. G is a 55-year-old man with a history of diabetes mellitus, coronary artery disease, hypertension, chronic low back pain secondary to degenerative joint disease, and substance use disorder admitted to the hospital for treatment of methicillin-sensitive *Staphylococcus aureus* (MSSA) bacteremia. Mr. G had been taking oxycodone as an outpatient for chronic pain and had been abstinent from use of intravenous drugs for several years prior to relapse 1 month before hospitalization. Mr. G recently lost his wife to cancer and attributed his relapse to this loss. After 6 days in the hospital, Mr. G reported increasing low back pain and requested an increase in pain medication. Diagnostic imaging of his back was negative for infectious complications. When told by the clinician that there was no imaging explanation for his increased pain, Mr. G suggested it was from the immobility and lack of sleep related to hospitalization. For several days, the clinician was in conflict with Mr. G over the issue of pain medication and accused him of "drug-seeking behavior." The clinician refused to increase the dose of pain medication which resulted in Mr. G requesting discharge from the hospital prior to outpatient parenteral antimicrobial treatment (OPAT) being arranged. The clinician performed an informed consent discussion and documented the risks and benefits of leaving the hospital, including death. Mr. G signed an AMA form prior to discharge, and no medications were prescribed at discharge in accordance with institutional policy. Mr. G was instructed to return to the hospital emergency department or to his primary care provider should he wish to be readmitted to continue treatment. Discharge instructions were for Mr. G to follow-up with his primary care provider in 1 week.

There are multiple cognitive and behavioral strategies that could have been used in an effort to prevent Mr. G from leaving the hospital AMA. This case demonstrates the lack of empathy commonly seen when interacting with patients with substance use disorder. In this patient population, medical teams often assume that patients are "drug seeking" when, in fact, they are often patients with a history of substance use, especially opioid use disorder, who may be suffering from unrecognized and, therefore, untreated withdrawal. In addition, Mr. G had recently lost a family member, so depression and sleep deprivation could have been contributing to his irritability and discomfort. Screening this patient for depression and requesting psychiatric consultation if clinically indicated, may have been beneficial. Pain is undertreated in patients with chronic opioid tolerance, and clinicians often feel uncomfortable increasing doses from baseline and/or prescribing the often very high doses required to effectively treat the pain. Appropriate consultation with pain medicine/addiction specialists and/or behavioral health professionals is imperative for this subset of patients. Ideally, these consultations should occur before a significant conflict or power struggle has developed between the patient and provider. Even if the patient is demonstrating "drug-seeking behavior", the overriding goal is still to convince the patient to remain in the hospital to complete therapy for his potentially life-threatening condition, and harm reduction strategies may well be needed to accomplish this goal. Involving other sources of support from family or friends, if available, would have also been a good strategy to help Mr. G remain in the hospital.

If efforts to mitigate the conflict between the clinician and Mr. G over pain medication are unsuccessful, consideration of alternative treatment plans should have been offered to him. Although oral antibiotics are not standard of care for MSSA bacteremia, individual clinicians may determine that they are a medically acceptable and reasonable alternative plan because the consequence of no therapy could be devastating for this patient. In this scenario, performance and documentation of a decisional capacity assessment and thorough informed consent discussion reflecting that the patient understands the consequences of his refusal of intravenous antibiotic therapy is indicated and is the most protective step the provider can take. Lastly, Mr. G should have been identified to the outpatient teams as a high priority for follow-up with emphasis on arranging ongoing intravenous antibiotic treatment as an outpatient if possible. Readmission should be offered if Mr. G changes his mind or his condition worsens after discharge and he agrees to hospitalization. The stigmatization of being discharged AMA should not preclude readmission if the patient subsequently agrees to treatment. These interventions would have been the preferred patient-centered approach to optimize care for Mr. G.

Case 2

Mr. R is a 45-year-old, with a history of tobacco and alcohol use disorder in remission, admitted to a university hospital for treatment of a brain abscess secondary to a bacterial infection. He is married with several children still living at home and had a daughter who is ill. Mr. R underwent uncomplicated neurosurgical drainage with subsequent recommendation for 6 weeks of intravenous (IV) antibiotic therapy. Mr. R was transferred back to his local hospital near his home after PICC line placement so that OPAT could be arranged. By the time he was transferred to his local hospital, Mr. R had already been hospitalized for 10 days. Mr. R arrived at his local hospital on a Friday evening and was informed that he would have to be admitted for the weekend for intravenous antibiotics because immediate OPAT could not be arranged until the following Monday. Mr. R expressed to the medical teams that he felt "lied to" about the discharge plan by the outside facility and requested to be discharged to home immediately. Prior to discharge, the inpatient provider contacted the infectious disease (ID), ethics, and psychiatry teams to assist with the case. Psychiatry determined that patient had decisional capacity and an informed consent discussion outlining the risks of leaving the hospital before completion of therapy was held with the patient. The ethics consultation service confirmed that a patient with decisional capacity has the right to accept or refuse any treatment. The option of giving the patient oral antibiotics until OPAT could be arranged was discussed with the ID team and considered as an alternative plan, but there was not an oral antibiotic option effective against the bacteria that would effectively cross the blood-brain barrier. The day after AMA discharge, the inpatient provider contacted the patient at home, who stated that he still wanted treatment with IV antibiotics. The patient explained that he left the hospital because his daughter was sick and needed him and he wanted to sleep in his own bed. The inpatient provider worked with the ID team and the emergency department (ED) physicians to arrange for the patient to come to the ED through the weekend for intravenous antibiotics. On Monday, the ID team arranged for an OPAT clinic appointment, outpatient therapy was arranged, and the patient ultimately completed treatment without interruption or complications.

We use this example to demonstrate a positive outcome in a similar case by utilizing some of the behavioral and cognitive strategies described above. Although the scenario of discharging a patient who clinically needs intravenous antibiotics but declines to remain in the hospital is similar, the provider's responses to the patient's request were very different. In this case, the healthcare teams did not argue or create a power struggle with Mr. R as they did with Mr. G, even though he arguably had an even higher risk of an adverse outcome if left untreated. The team in the second case involved appropriate consultants when the patient first declined to remain in the hospital, especially given this high-risk clinical scenario. Psychiatry was consulted to perform the decisional capacity assessment as this case involved refusal of a relatively low-risk treatment with a high clinical benefit and the bar for ensuring decisional capacity was very high. Mr. R's healthcare teams acknowledged and apologized for the miscommunication which was a positive way to demonstrate empathy for this patient. They then employed motivational interviewing to gain greater insight into the patient's motives for leaving the hospital and to generate motivation for the patient to participate in treatment planning. Mr. R clearly had competing family obligations but still wanted treatment and understood the consequences of not completing therapy. The primary and consulting teams worked together to come up with an alternative plan of care so that the patient could receive antibiotics through the weekend until OPAT could be arranged. Some of the teams involved were rightly concerned that this alternative care plan would set a difficult precedent for the hospital and issues of liability were raised. Although these concerns are understandable, it is important to remember that the overall rate of AMA discharge is only 1–2% of all hospital admissions, and the ethical and clinical analysis of each case should be conducted independently. For this type of high-risk medical condition, one can argue that it was reasonable for the healthcare system to accommodate this patient, even though it was not the standard protocol for the facility.

Case 3

Mrs. J is a 73-year-old with hypertension, diabetes, and chronic obstructive pulmonary disease with baseline home oxygen requirement of 2 l/min admitted for community acquired pneumonia. On day 2 of hospitalization, Mrs. J remained febrile with a persistent leukocytosis and 5 l/min oxygen requirement. She stated that she must leave the hospital because there is no one to help her walk and feed her dog who is home alone. The provider advised the patient that she "might die" if she leaves the hospital and tried to persuade the patient that her best chance to provide ongoing care for her dog is to stay in the hospital until she is well enough to return home. The provider does not want to provide oral antibiotics or arrange for home oxygen and does not feel obligated to do so since Mrs. J is leaving AMA. The patient signs the AMA form and is discharged to home.

This is a common scenario where several interventions could be useful. Caring for a companion animal is a common reason that patients request to leave the hospital before completion of recommended therapy. Utilizing other sources of family/ friend or local organizational support to assist this patient in caring for her beloved dog would show compassion and commitment to the patient's holistic welfare. Social work assistance would also be beneficial to assist the patient in locating friends or relatives that might be able to help to care for the dog until Mrs. J is ready for discharge. Providers often fear being liable for adverse outcomes when patients do not follow recommendations. This case demonstrates a common misperception that providing oral medication or arranging for home oxygen increases liability for physicians when, in fact, there may be far more liability for not providing these therapies when they are clinically indicated. Such potential responsibility is even greater when withholding the treatment could do grave harm to the patient. The common belief that an AMA form absolves the provider from liability from adverse outcomes is not well supported and is certainly not protective when the patient is denied otherwise clinically indicated care.

Operational Strategies

We will now briefly describe efforts at one institution to operationalize some of these strategies for AMA discharge using a quality improvement systems redesign strategy. This effort was designed to promote a just culture in which the AMA discharge was viewed as a unique type of transition of care that should be optimized for patient safety, rather than as a purely risk management event where both providers and patients are to blame.

Facilities can work to improve the culture surrounding an AMA discharge by offering providers tools and guidelines to support them in optimizing the transition of care to the outpatient setting should patients choose to leave AMA. Recent efforts at one facility to operationalize the best practice elements of an AMA discharge described above resulted in improved performance and documentation of these elements [26]. This excerpt, written by a registered nurse interviewed on the process improvement team, describes the challenges of an AMA discharge:

> Situations like these are very stressful for the nurse, physician and patient. In my experience, when the patient is cognitively intact and has made the decision to leave, there is not much that we can do to change their mind. Often, there are only a few minutes to act and at times it is difficult to have the AMA form signed by the patient at all. From my perspective, standard guidelines regarding patients leaving AMA would assist staff during the limited amount of time available with the patient. These guidelines should include a *checklist* of items that need to be completed or asked prior to a patient leaving AMA. The items on the checklist should be clear, concise and easy to understand.

The process embraced the concepts of shared decision-making, assessment and documentation of decisional capacity, informed consent, and eliminating the use of AMA forms with emphasis on optimizing the transition of care to the outpatient setting. The following 11 elements were identified as the foundation of a best practice for an AMA discharge:

1. Assessment and documentation of decisional capacity
2. Documentation of informed consent discussion
3. Medication counseling documented
4. Patient advised to return to hospital/emergency department if indicated
5. Documentation of line removal
6. Discharge instructions provided
7. Provider notification by nursing staff
8. Transportation assistance offered to patient
9. Nursing documentation of AMA discharge
10. Nursing supervisor notification of AMA discharge
11. Electronic patient event report (ePER) completed

To establish baseline compliance with performance and documentation of the best practice elements, a retrospective chart review of fiscal year 2014 AMA data was completed. A total of 66 AMA discharges occurred during this period. This review demonstrated that there were significant opportunities for process improvement. Complimentary electronic medical record note templates were created for both providers and nursing staff, prompting them to perform these best practice elements. The provider note focused on assessment and documentation of decisional capacity, informed consent, and outcome of discussion with patient. Providers were encouraged to prescribe medications when appropriate. The nursing note functioned as a checklist to optimize patient safety prior to AMA discharge. This checklist focused on provider and supervisor notification, line removal, equipment needs, social work assistance, provision of discharge instructions, and completion of a patient event report. In this process, the patient event report is sent to the patient safety coordinator and primary care team. When alerted, the primary care team can prioritize appropriate post-acute care, and the patient safety coordinator can further investigate any systems issues related to the discharge. Both electronic note templates use prompts and standardized text to improve ease of practice and compliance with the use of the templates.

After baseline data was collected, a 3-month pilot study looked at 16 AMA events and revealed that compliance with performance and documentation of the 11 best practice elements increased dramatically across all domains. The improvement can be seen in Fig. 7.2, which compares the baseline and pilot data [26].

This systems redesign offered care teams practical tools to guide them through the AMA discharge process. Key to the successful transformation of the approach to AMA was collaboration and communication between nurses and physicians toward the goal of patient safety, rather than conflict and blame that often accompanies AMA discharges. The process improvement team engaged hospital leadership

Fig. 7.2 Compliance with performance of best practice elements of an AMA discharge. This graph shows the change in compliance rate of performance and documentation of the 11 best practice elements identified for an AMA discharge. Significant increase in rate of compliance for pilot data is demonstrated

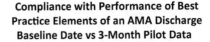
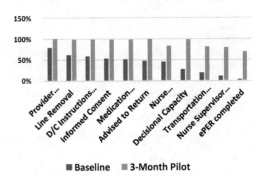

who promoted a just culture in which the AMA discharge was viewed as a unique type of transition of care that should be optimized for patient safety, rather than as a risk management event where both providers and patients may feel blamed.

Although small in number of patients, the pilot study demonstrated that by using a quality improvement systems redesign strategy, a hospital can improve performance and documentation of the best practice elements for an AMA discharge. Because there are such differences in provider education and comfort levels with AMA discharge, future efforts should be directed at studying translational approaches that assist care teams in managing an AMA discharge and its effect on patient outcomes.

Conclusion

In this chapter, we have discussed many of the evidence-based best practices and associated cognitive and behavioral strategies for the management of AMA discharges. Patients who are discharged from the hospital AMA represent a very high-risk cohort in terms of morbidity, mortality, readmission, and healthcare resource utilization. Bioethicists and hospital risk managers are increasingly recognizing that AMA discharge should be treated as a unique transition of care that should be optimized for patient safety. We reviewed the literature and analyzed some of the common barriers and misconceptions that may lead providers to pursue an AMA discharge. We also discussed the patient-centered strategies and concepts of shared decision-making, motivational interviewing, and behavioral and cognitive techniques and suggested operational tools and processes to assist providers in negotiating a more productive health outcome for patients who request AMA discharge.

References

1. Daniels RS, Margolis PM, Carson RC. Hospital discharges against medical advice: origin and prevention. Arch Gen Psychiatry. 1963;8:30–40.
2. Schlauch RW, Reich P, Kelly MJ. Leaving the hospital against medical advice. N Engl J Med. 1979;300:22–4.
3. Fiscella K, Meldrum S, Barnett S. Hospital discharge against advice after myocardial infarction: deaths and readmissions. Am J Med. 2007;120:1047–53.
4. Hwang SW, Li J, Gupta R, Chien V, Martin RE. What happens to patients who leave hospital against medical advice? CMAJ. 2003;168(4):417–20.
5. Ibrahim SA, Kwoh CK, Krishnan E. Factors associated with patients who leave acute-care hospitals against medical advice. Am J Public Health. 2007;97(12):2204–8.
6. Alfandre DJ. "I'm going home": discharges against medical advice. Mayo Clin Proc. 2009;84(3):255–60.
7. Kraut A, Fransoo R, Olafson K, Ramsey CD, Yogendran M, Garland A. A population-based analysis of leaving the hospital against medical advice: incidence and associated variables. BMC Health Serv Res. 2013;13:415–24.
8. Lekas HM, Alfandre D, Gordon P, Harwood K, Yin MT. The role of patient-provider interactions: using an accounts framework to explain hospital discharges against medical advice. Soc Sci Med. 2016;156:106–13. https://doi.org/10.1016/j.socscimed.2016.03.018.
9. Glasgow JM, Vaughn-Sarrazin M, Kaboli PJ. Leaving against medical advice (AMA): risk of 30-day mortality and hospital readmission. J Gen Intern Med. 2010;25(9):926–9.
10. Southern WN, Nahvi S, Arnsten JH. Increased risk of mortality and readmission among patients discharged against medical advice. Am J Med. 2012;125(6):594–602.
11. Garland A, Ramsey CD, Fransoo R, Olafson K, Chateau D, Yogendran M, Kraut A. Rates of readmission and death associated with leaving hospital against medical advice: a population-based study. CMAJ. 2013;185(14):1207–14.
12. Alfandre D. Reconsidering against medical advice discharges: embracing patient-centeredness to promote high quality care and a renewed research agenda. J Gen Intern Med. 2013;28(12):1657–62.
13. Spooner KK, Salemi JL, Salihu HM, Zoorob RJ. Discharge against medical advice in the United States, 2002–2011. Mayo Clin Proc. 2017;92(4):525–35.
14. Alfandre D. Clinical recommendations in medical practice: a proposed framework to reduce bias and improve the quality of medical decisions. J Clin Ethics. 2016;27(1):21–7.
15. Appelbaum PS. Assessment of patients' competence to consent to treatment. N Engl J Med. 2007;357:1834–40.
16. Devitt PJ, Devitt AC, Dewan M. An examination of whether discharging patients against medical advice protects physicians from malpractice charges. Psychiatr Serv. 2000;51(7):899–902.
17. Devitt PJ, Devitt AC, Dewan M. Does identifying a discharge as "Against Medical Advice" confer legal protection? J Fam Pract. 2000;49(3):224–7.
18. Ganzini L, Volicer L, Nelson WA, Fox E, Derse AR. Ten myths of decision-making capacity. J Am Med Dir Assoc. 2005;6:S100–4. https://doi.org/10.1016/j.jamda.2005.03.021.
19. Wigder HN, Leslie K, Mathew A. Insurance companies refusing payment for patients who leave the emergency department against medical advice is a myth. Ann Emerg Med. 2010;55(4):393.
20. Schaefer GR, Matus H, Schumann JH, Sauter K, Vekhter B, Meltzer DO, Arora VM. Financial responsibility of hospitalized patients who left against medical advice: medical urban legend? J Gen Intern Med. 2012;27(7):825–30.
21. Berger JT. Discharge against medical advice: ethical considerations and professional obligations. J Hosp Med. 2008;3:403–8.
22. Quill TE, Cassell CK. Nonabandonment: a central obligation for physicians. Ann Intern Med. 1995;122:368–74.

23. Clark MA, Abbott JT, Adyanthaya T. Ethics seminars: a best-practice approach to navigating the against-medical-advice discharge. Acad Emerg Med. 2014;21:1050–7.
24. Alfandre D. What is wrong with discharges against medical advice (and how to fix them). JAMA. 2013;310(22):2393–4.
25. Karasz A, Dyche L, Selwyn P. Physicians' experiences of caring for late-stage HIV patients in the post-HAART era: challenges and adaptations. Soc Sci Med. 2003;57(9):1609–20.
26. Fleming H, Tryon C, Gresham T, Olson DS. Creating a best practice for discharges against medical advice. J Hosp Med. 2016;11(suppl 1). http://shmabstracts.com/abstract/creating-a-best-practice-for-discharges-against-medical-advice/. Accessed 17 Mar 2016.

Chapter 8
Against Medical Advice Discharges from the Emergency Department

Jay M. Brenner and Thomas E. Robey

AMA Discharges from the Emergency Department

The emergency department presents a unique context for patients leaving the acute care setting against medical advice (AMA), and experience from emergency providers may help other areas of the health-care system address the ongoing challenge of increasing prevalence of AMA. It is important to distinguish the types of self-discharges from the emergency department (ED), as well as the differences between capacity determination in the acute and undifferentiated context of the ED versus other care settings. The regularity of intoxicated, aggressive, and sometimes uncooperative patients in the ED provides a foundation for improving care for patients discharged AMA but also for minimizing other types of departures before completion of a medical episode of care. Just as no patient's disease presents the same way, there is no one-size-fits-all approach to the AMA discharge. We describe three cases to illustrate the central aspects of the AMA challenge with analysis to follow that will clarify the risks and best practices of discharging patients AMA from the ED.

J. M. Brenner (✉)
Department of Emergency Medicine, Upstate Medical University, Syracuse, NY, USA
e-mail: brennerj@upstate.edu

T. E. Robey
Elson S. Floyd College of Medicine, Washington State University, Everett, WA, USA

Emergency Department, Providence Regional Medical Center, Everett, WA, USA

North Sound Emergency Medicine, Everett, WA, USA

© Springer International Publishing AG, part of Springer Nature 2018
D. Alfandre (ed.), *Against-Medical-Advice Discharges from the Hospital*,
https://doi.org/10.1007/978-3-319-75130-6_8

Cases

Case 1: Precious

Frank Strong (pseudonym) is a 66-year-old retired widower who lives at home with his Irish terrier, Precious. He came to the ED this evening after 3 days of worsening non-specific abdominal pain that migrated to the right lower quadrant. His physical exam and initial labs suggested appendicitis, and a CT scan confirmed a swollen inflamed appendix without rupture. After you relay the diagnosis, prognosis, and treatment options, Mr. Strong indicates that he understands the need for emergent surgery but refuses to undergo surgery tonight, opting instead to return tomorrow for the procedure. He even repeats the possibility of rupture and the mortality associated with rupture. "But doc, there's no one to take care of Precious tonight." He promises to come back tomorrow, "or else you can come pick me up."

Case 2: Smoke 'Em if You Got 'Em

Tien Do (pseudonym) is a 26-year-old second-generation Vietnamese-American woman who comes in with her boyfriend, Jackson, because of dehydration from intractable vomiting. She hasn't been able to keep fluids down for 3 days. She says that when she loses her appetite, she smokes extra marijuana because that usually makes her hungry. Since being in the waiting room, she has been dry heaving and continues to do so when you interview her. "Doctor, usually they give me d- d-Dilaudid for my horrible stomach pain, and Zofran never works. You need to use Phenergan and possibly Benadryl." You share your thoughts about this being cyclic vomiting or marijuana hyperemesis syndrome, but Ms. Do notes that unless you give her the medicines she prefers, she plans on leaving.

Case 3: "Come on, Guys!"

Hector Jones (pseudonym) is a familiar face around the emergency department. He's often found on the village green minimally responsive, intoxicated by alcohol, and with poor hygiene. Not known for courtesy, he is regularly and efficiently managed by the ED staff because he rarely makes a scene and doesn't argue when he's discharged from the department come morning. He doesn't want to quit drinking and does have a history of withdrawal. This evening, he was found down and arrived by ambulance with police escort due to his agitation. He has a new abrasion on his forehead and a dried bloody nose. Hector recognizes you and the nurses and while being held down by restraints pleads, "Come on guys! You know I just need to get my liquor so I don't withdraw." He wants to be discharged, as usual. The officers roll their eyes and the medics leave promptly.

Definitions

Several definitions need clarification before delving further into the discussion of what is classically referred to as patients leaving against medical advice (AMA) from the ED. As with other areas of medical care, AMA discharge has been used broadly to describe any instance of a patient leaving before he or she is officially discharged by the care provider. A closer examination reveals that such a broad description is inadequate in the ED and that other incomplete medical visits, when patients leave without completing treatment, should be added and further divided into the following categories: left without being seen (LWBS), left without being triaged (LWBT), leaving without being discharged (LWBD), and AMA discharges. These three types of patient departures, where patients leave without completing treatment, are more common than AMA discharges. With each category of departure, the dynamics of the patient-physician relationship should be considered.

LWBS occurs when a patient presents to the emergency department and leaves before seeing a physician or advanced practice clinician (APC – which includes nurse practitioners and physician assistants). LWBS is a common quality metric that measures access and can be included on an emergency department's daily dashboard reviewed by department and hospital leadership. LWBS can be used to describe a broad range of scenarios, depending on which point in the encounter the patient leaves. Patients may leave before even registering with the front desk or administration; in this situation, there is no record of the patient's presence in the ED. More commonly, a patient might have registered but left without being triaged (LWBT), or the patient was triaged but left before being roomed or seen by the definitive care provider (physician or APC). Classically, LWBS is used to describe patients who leave before coming in contact with the definitive care provider who is responsible for their care. There is no patient-physician relationship with LWBS or LWBT.

LWBD describes the patient who is not formally dispositioned and discharged by the care provider. There is a patient-physician relationship here, but it is not concluded mutually. The physician or provider does not have the opportunity to communicate risk of departure. The colloquial term for this, when exiting the medical facility without notifying anyone, is *elopement* or that the *patient eloped*.

AMA discharge occurs when the patient leaves the medical facility contrary to the medical team's recommendations and can be applied regardless of whether a patient signs any specific AMA forms. Recently, this definition has been applied specifically to differentiate it from the abovementioned definitions. A discharge should be considered AMA only when the patient discusses their care plan with their provider as part of an informed consent discussion and then chooses to leave despite the provider's recommendations. This is a crucial differentiation between AMA discharge and elopement/LWBD, LWBT, or LWBS because there is an opportunity for an informed consent discussion between the patient and their provider in a functional patient-physician relationship.

Review of Existing Literature

There is a sizeable literature on patients leaving without completing treatment. The literature covers the medical, legal, and ethical considerations related to these issues. National estimates of patients leaving AMA are consistently between 1% and 2% [1, 2], and the number and proportion have been on the rise. Separate measures of national LWBS rates indicate an additional 2% of patients leave without receiving or completing treatment [4]. In 1995, an estimated 1.1 million (1.41% of total) patients left prematurely; but this number was 2.1 million (1.92% of total visits) in 2002 [7].

According to the patients themselves, the two most frequent reasons for why they left AMA from the ED are perceiving that they are waiting too long for care and not wanting to pay the co-pay [9]. Interestingly, over 90% of patients in one particular study were triaged within 30 min of coming in, but 60% of those patients still responded that they left because they were waiting too long [9], pointing to delays between triage and provider contact as a reason for leaving. It is important not to conflate AMA with the LWBT/LWBS/LWBD categories because (1) the nature of the patient experience is different, (2) the nature of communicated risk is different, and (3) the strategies to mitigate each type of departure are vastly different. Of those who leave early (AMA or LWBD), many of those patients come back to the emergency department (ED) with the same chief complaint or go to be evaluated elsewhere for the same issue within a week or two [1, 3, 8].

Factors that increase the odds of a patient leaving before being seen include having government insurance (Medicaid, Medicare, etc.), coming to the ED when the department is at or over capacity, seeking care at a larger urban medical center, and being of African-American or Hispanic race [2]. One study noted that patients were more likely to leave early if the ED capacity was at 100% with the most pronounced effect was seen at ED capacity of over 140% [5]. One-third of the patients who leave prematurely continue to have symptoms in the days after their incomplete visit [3]. The most common categories of chief complaints for these patients vary in nature and potential severity: ranging from cardiovascular, respiratory, or abdominal symptoms to musculoskeletal pain [3, 4] and mirror the typical reasons for all presentations. One study reinforces a generally accepted notion that patients who LWBS were more likely to be of low triage acuity and that ED treatment may not have been needed [4].

Pediatric patient encounters have separate risk factors and complaints related to leaving AMA or LWBS. Factors that increase the odds for pediatric visits ending with AMA or LWBS include age over 15 years, self-registration without a parent, visit involving a consultant, arrival by ambulance, and a chief complaint of abdominal pain [6]. Negative risk factors (i.e., factors that would make a patient leave AMA less likely) for pediatric patients included urgent triage, diagnosis of infection, and diseases of the nervous system, sense organs, or respiratory tract [6]. For pediatric patients, in particular, determination of child safety and notification to child protective services for selective AMA discharges is discussed in Chap. 10.

Other literature addresses the issue of incomplete or inadequate documentation of AMA and LWBS discharges. Apart from the clinical or administrative information gaps inherent in a patient leaving before completing treatment, the content and quality of documentation of the departure varies widely. To address this, some hospitals have adopted AMA forms requiring patient signatures before leaving. These are variable in the detail of further care instructions and typically have boiler plate legal language with few lines for case-specific information to be completed by a provider or nurse. Studies have shown repeatedly that those forms are often left incomplete and, in case of a lawsuit, are not a sufficient defense [1] without accompanying medical chart documentation. Within the literature, there is a general consensus that AMA forms, even if signed by the patient, do not substitute for thorough and relevant documentation, nor are they an excuse for not providing otherwise medically indicated care. Furthermore, AMA forms themselves are not a sufficient release of physician or hospital liability.

There is a general consensus that clear documentation of a thorough discussion with patients will provide the desired legal protection, even if the patient refuses treatment or wants to leave before the visit is complete. Clark et al. proposes the AIMED (assess, investigate, mitigate, explain, document) model to achieve these goals [1], and this model is useful in an emergency department setting (Table 8.1). The *assess* step determines whether the patient has the capacity to refuse or agree to treatment. Patients in the ED may be severely sick, mentally ill, or under the influence of drugs or alcohol. It is critical in an AMA discharge to assess whether the patient can engage in a rational discussion and provide informed consent, or whether the patient may require treatment against his or her will, and whether the incapacitation is likely to be transient. Disagreement with a provider's plan does not by itself make a patient lack decision-making capacity or incapable of making a treatment decision. The *investigate* step identifies the patient's reasons for leaving. Some reasons that a patient may want to leave a treatment facility early include inadequate comfort, poor communication by the staff, withdrawal symptoms, or pressing family or work matters. Enlisting the help of friends and family to gather information and work out a plan that may be more acceptable to the patient is useful in this step. The *mitigate* step attempts to provide the best care possible, even if the patient does not want to stay. Examples of this include giving initial medicine doses in the ED and prescribing oral antibiotics or giving the patient a referral to a primary care doctor and arranging for staff to call and check in with the patient. The objective here is one of harm reduction, to provide maximum care possible while respecting the patient's autonomy, even if the patient is not willing to follow the optimal health-promoting treatment plan presented. This process aims to optimize the patient's care and promote his health within the identified constraints. The *explain* step reiterates the best treatment plan within the identified constraints, as well as alternative treatment options, should the patient wish to leave or disagree with the initial plan. This step should also serve to provide the patient with thorough discharge instructions and an assurance that the patient is welcome to return to the ED for any reason. The *document* step is to assure good record keeping. The ideal note should objectively describe (1) any medical care provided, (2) the circumstances leading to

Table 8.1 A practical
approach: AIMED

Assess	Severity of illness/urgency of treatment
	Decision-making capacity (treat underlying cause if impaired)
	Degree of risk to patient's health and welfare
Investigate	Patient's reason for leaving
	Comfort (symptom management)
	Communication regarding care plan
	Withdrawal syndromes
	Pressing responsibilities like child, elder, or pet care issues
	Allies such as primary care provider or family member
Mitigate	Offer maximal necessary treatment acceptable to patient
	Provide prescriptions for medications as indicated
	Provide optimal follow-up plan and discharge instructions
Explain	Original treatment plan risks and benefits
	Specific dangers of failing to follow proposed plan
	Alternative plan
	Discharge instructions including reasons to return
	That the patient is welcome to return at any time
Document	Medical screening exam
	Decision-making capacity assessment
	Discussion of initial treatment offered
	Discussion of patient refusal and reasoning
	Efforts to negotiate, recruit family/ friends
	Alternative plan with risks and benefits
	Discharge instructions including when to return
	Efforts to locate if no discharge conversation occurred

the patient's preference in leaving, (3) an assessment of patient's decision-making capacity if appropriate, (4) the discussion of the risks and benefits of the recommended and alternative treatment plans, and finally (5) detailed discharge instructions.

As emergency departments are more overcrowded, more patients may wish to leave before treatment is completed, and many of these patients continue to suffer from the same issues and often return to the ED or seek care elsewhere within days of the initial presentation. In general practice, the patient who returns after an AMA discharge may experience stereotyped perceptions and the stigma of having been "AMA." Most of the discussion surrounding AMA discharge has been centered on legal protection, but the ethical issues surrounding patients discharged AMA should also address the negative attitudes associated with it. Further awareness of the pitfalls of AMA discharge should be applied to large, urban medical centers or those with increased proportion of underserved patients. Despite attempts to mitigate risk with strategies detailed below, AMA continues to be a source of legal and ethical concern. This reality should not leave the reader with a sense of hopelessness, rather it should motivate the astute clinician to invest in a therapeutic relationship with a patient and address a patient's request to leave with care and detail. In summary, the patient encounter should include treatments to minimize stigma and patient risk, maximize the likelihood of follow-up, and offer the best alternatives that still promote the patient's health, all within an honest and professional patient-physician relationship.

Myths

Our experience is that as much myth and stigma is applied by providers to the issue of AMA as to other stereotyped conditions in medicine. As with preconceived notions of substance abuse, intimate partner violence, and psychiatric disease, it is important to be aware of the myths and common practices in order not to let them interfere with professionalism and high-quality compassionate care. Providers with an accurate understanding of the issue are well positioned to reduce legal and ethical hazards associated with AMA discharge.

Using a best practice approach such as AIMED to minimize patient risk and maximize likelihood of follow-up is central to an optimal AMA discharge. Separate from this, it is unfortunately common to designate a patient who refuses recommended treatment and is leaving the ED with the moniker "AMA." Though it could be appropriate for a patient who returns to the ED after leaving AMA the day before to be described in the clinical note as, "Mr. X, who left AMA for the same complaint yesterday, returns to the ED requesting further care," it may not provide relevant clinical information to have the AMA element as the primary descriptor in the chart's opening sentence. In addition, when the patient expresses an intention to leave, the care team often will cognitively convert the request into the verb "the patient wants to AMA."

Insurance

Some emergency providers may indicate that a patient's visit will not be covered by insurance in order to leverage the patient to agree to stay for further treatment. In one study of all ED providers, 57% believed that insurers will not reimburse ED visits when patients leave AMA. When systematically evaluated, 19 insurance companies, including HMOs, PPOs, Medicare, Medicaid, and worker's compensation, fully reimbursed all of the visits where the patient left AMA [10]. It is therefore both misleading and potentially coercive to threaten patients to stay for further treatment under the guise of their insurer not covering their visit if they request to leave.

Liability

Many emergency providers believe that an AMA discharge can protect them from liability in a medical malpractice action and that such a discharge requires an AMA form. Levy et al. argue that signing out a patient AMA may terminate a physician's legal duty to treat. An AMA discharge may create an assumption of risk defense, and evidence of the patient's refusal of care and assumption of risk in the medical record removes any later claim that they did not know the risks of leaving. The same authors, however, argue that "an AMA form is not required for proper documentation." Case law has demonstrated that AMA forms and institutional procedures do not completely insulate emergency physicians from liability [11]. This raises the obvious question that if such a form is neither necessary, nor completely protective, then why is it used?

Similar to the threat of nonpayment by insurance companies, some emergency providers may use the form to persuade patients to stay for further treatment under the assumption that the patient may not have legal recourse in case of a tort if they sign the form. However, the patient may litigate regardless of their AMA status. A patient frustrated by the designation of leaving AMA and having to sign a form acknowledging such risk may be more likely to sue.

Medications

It is important to clarify whether, in requesting to leave, the patient is refusing all treatment, since often, he or she is only refusing the treatment plan that the clinician offered. As a result, some health-care providers are reluctant to prescribe medications or schedule follow-up appointments for patients requesting to leave. In one study, 36% of inpatient nurses believed that patients should not receive medications and follow-up because of leaving AMA, and 6% of attending physicians and 16% of resident physicians believed the same [12]. For the sake of improving health outcomes, patients should receive clinically indicated medications and follow-up even if they request to leave. Not providing a second-best option of prescriptions and follow-up appointment in order to persuade patients to stay may be coercive because it appears to be a threat of penalty upon refusal of recommended care. If done in order to punish patients, the action could be considered abusive and unprofessional. In order to improve care, mitigate patient risk, and maximize likelihood of follow-up, emergency providers should prescribe all indicated medications and provide any reasonable alternative to the recommended treatment plan when a patient leaves AMA.

Observation

There is an increasing prevalence of AMA discharges after patients are notified of their admission status as observation. Observation is a relatively new category of admission driven by expectations by insurance payers that patients with certain conditions (most commonly, low-risk chest pain, syncope, or transient ischemic attack) can be evaluated in a 1-day inpatient stay. Though insurance coverage is changing, these stays are often not fully covered by some payers, leaving patients with a higher proportion of the cost of admission. Frequently, these patients have multiple comorbidities and are taking many medications, the administration of which will not be covered during their hospital stay because of the observation status. The reason for admission, however, may not qualify them for inpatient status, due to decisions made by the admitting team. The emergency provider may be frustrated by this dilemma especially when it occurs near the tail end of their provision of care. When the observation status comes as a surprise, it frequently upsets the patient who has already agreed to admission but may not be able to afford the financial costs of an observation stay. It is a myth that inpatients cannot be downgraded to or upgraded from observation status upon further review.

Procedures

Occasionally, a patient may refuse a recommended procedure as part of a diagnostic evaluation. For example, a patient with severe headache and a normal CT brain scan may decline a lumbar puncture needed to rule out a subtle subarachnoid hemorrhage (SAH). The patient's justification is often to avoid undesired discomfort with the procedure. She may acknowledge the slight risk of missed SAH; however, she values the benefit of avoiding the potential pain from a spinal needle. ED providers frequently label such a patient who declines a recommended diagnostic procedure as AMA and have them sign an AMA form. This practice can be ethically problematic. It is generally sufficient to report the discussion of the risks and benefits of the procedure and the alternatives (including no treatment), the patient's reasons for declining, and a decision-making capacity assessment. This serves as good evidence of an informed consent discussion and need not undergo an AMA process.

Legal Considerations in the ED

Although the primary consideration in managing patients leaving AMA from the emergency department should always be an ethical provision of medical care, there are legal implications to this decision that the emergency medical provider should be aware. Central to the concept of patient refusal of treatment is the importance of establishing capacity. When determining capacity both legal criteria (age over 18 or minor emancipation) and clinical capacity criteria must be met. A good test of clinical capacity is the patient's ability to understand and state back his or her medical condition, treatment options, and risks and benefits of the treatment options. The patient's ability to do this is dependent on the medical provider providing an informed discussion of refusal so that patients are able to have the information to make an informed decision. Physicians may be sued for allowing patients to leave AMA or for treating patients who are declining treatment. The best defense against these lawsuits is a thorough informed consent conversation with patients as accompanied by clear documentation of the treatment refusal conversation. Alternatively, clear evidence as to why a patient is being treated against his or her wishes must also be documented. Clinical capacity evaluation need not be performed by a psychiatric provider but may be useful if mandating emergency treatment over objection or if a patient suffers from a serious mental illness and lacks decisional capacity [13]. Likewise, AMA in the setting of questionable capacity could be further supported by a second provider's assessment, including input from a mental health professional.

Most litigation regarding AMA discharges surrounds inadequate transmission of medical information to patients, resulting in unformed patient decisions. To make an informed decision, patients must understand the provided information regarding all treatment options, benefits of these options, as well as risks of not pursuing them. The specific risks of leaving AMA should be explained clearly and documented. Although the emergency provider may feel compelled to argue the importance of the proposed medical treatment a patient is declining, there have been cases where emergency providers have been liable for exaggerating risks of refusing care in the manner described above in the Myths section. Furthermore, despite a patient being discharged AMA, emergency providers must continue to treat the patient within the identified constraints and provide them with clinically appropriate medications and follow-up referrals or information. For instance, a patient declining an abscess incision and drainage with evidence of surrounding cellulitis may still requires or benefit from an oral antibiotic prescription even if the benefit is minimized compared to if the patient agreed to the incision and drainage. Failure to provide medically appropriate care in this situation can lead to legal liability, even if proper documentation of AMA is provided to the patient and in the medical record [14].

A legal requirement unique to the ED and consultants to the ED that complicates AMA discharges is the Emergency Medical Treatment and Active Labor Act (EMTALA). EMTALA was passed in 1986 as an unfunded mandate requiring anyone presenting to a Medicare-participating hospital or emergency department be evaluated and stabilized regardless of insurance status or ability to pay. The federal government was responding to multiple complaints of private hospitals dumping patients without insurance to public hospitals leading to untoward patient outcomes. Violations of EMTALA result in significant penalties including hospital fines of up to $50,000 per violation, physician fines, or termination of the hospital or physician's Medicare provider agreement. It is a requirement that emergency providers evaluate all patients arriving to the ED and that if a patient needs transfer to a different hospital, that receiving facility has the capacity to care for the transferred patient. EMTALA relates to the AMA discharge when the patient reports an inability to pay as the reason to leave OR when the patient states an intention to go to a different hospital. To fulfill the intent of EMTALA, it is recommended that patients who would like to leave the emergency department AMA due to inability to pay are specifically encouraged to stay by minimizing financial concerns by involving social work or charity care. It may be considered a violation of EMTALA directly, or the spirit of EMTALA, by providing information about cost of care without encouraging patients to remain for treatment. Due to the high penalties of violating EMTALA and increased scrutiny by regulatory agencies, hospitals strive to not only avoid EMTALA violations but also the appearance of them. Likewise, providers should take care not to recommend a patient seek care after an AMA discharge at a different but equivalent medical facility, as this could violate EMTALA's antidumping statute. An appropriate plan includes recommendations to "return to this or any other medical facility to seek further care." If there is concern for potential EMTALA violation, the AMA conversation needs thorough documentation, and signed or unsigned paperwork should be retained [15].

While institutional AMA documentation does not eliminate the risk of litigation, it may increase the burden on the plaintiff to establish malpractice in the case of a legal action. The paperwork attempts to make an official termination of the physician's legal duty to treat and is suggested that it protects against claims of EMTALA violations. Paperwork, in combination with a documented conversation, establishes that a patient who chooses to leave AMA voluntarily takes on the risk of any negative consequences and the patient assumes the responsibility to seek further care and increases the burden on the plaintiff to claim they were never made aware of the risks of leaving AMA.

General Approaches to AMA Discharges in the ED

There is no single approach to the AMA discharge from the emergency department. Two components of an AMA discharge should be addressed: the medical management of the patient and the legal risk to the health-care provider(s) and their institution.

Many authors have proposed strategies addressing the legal risk, most notably Clark et al., including patients signing specific forms when leaving AMA [11, 13] and physicians carefully documenting conversations with the patient in the medical record [1, 12]. In general, we recommend an approach similar to Clark et al.'s AIMED (assess, investigate, mitigate, explain, document) [1]. In addition to this, hospital systems also include AMA options in EMRs and will indicate AMA as a discharge category. However, recent data sheds light on the use of EMRs and AMA discharges. A recent survey of emergency physicians and nurse practitioners regarding their reactions to patients requesting to leave uncovered that a reason to designate a patient AMA and have them sign an AMA form was facilitated by using the electronic medical record (EMR) [16]. Certainly, an EMR can be helpful to document statistics regarding rates of patients leaving AMA, leaving without being seen, leaving without being triaged, or leaving without being discharged. However, one study which examined the rate of patients leaving without treatment did not find a difference between the use of an EMR and a paper system. Suffice it to say, the EMR did not affect this rate [17]. While an EMR may provide a tool to document and track patients requesting to leave, it in itself is not a good reason to designate a patient as AMA or coerce them into signing a form. Some systems require a specific protocol for each AMA discharge. The emphasis on legal risk and documentation thought shouldn't overshadow the primary component of an AMA discharge: the medical management of the patient in refusing treatment or leaving without treatment completion.

A one-size-fits-all strategy has the potential to overlook an individual patient's specific needs to optimize health outcomes. The growing attention to shared decision-making in medicine has a role in informing the approach to AMA discharges. We propose three categories of management for AMA discharges, each addressing the legal risk and medical management. Providers can be *persuasive*, *permissive*, or *paternalistic* (or a combination of all three) when faced with an AMA discharge situation. The *persuasive* approach builds upon the rapport developed between the provider and patient and results in a middle ground treatment plan that reduces risk but may not be the physician's first recommended course. The *permissive* AMA discharge occurs at the conclusion of a shared decision-making process when the provider acknowledges the inability to convince the patient to follow an ideal or compromise treatment plan but acknowledges the patient's right to refuse the recommendations. The *paternalistic* approach to AMA discharge relies on the physician making a decision in the incapacitated patient's best interest when there is emergency treatment needed and no surrogate decision-maker is available.

Persuasive and permissive approaches rely on the patient having full capacity to make medical decisions. The rapport between patient and provider in the ED will often dictate the direction between the persuasive and permissive AMA discharges. Creative problem-solving, including compromises that may run against providers' professional principles and values, may go far in preventing an unsafe discharge. Emergency physicians are well-familiar with the chain-smoking patient who wants to sneak a cigarette before admission. Addressing the nicotine dependence may be the only obstacle to convincing a patient to undergo testing or treatment for her condition. Two persuasive approaches would be (1) to weigh the risks of "one last cigarette" against hospital policy and let the patient smoke before admission or (2) more ideally to seize on the patient's nascent wish to quit smoking and perform a brief negotiated interview and provide nicotine replacement. Involving family and friends is a useful technique for persuasion, especially for certain groups of patients. Another example of persuasive treatment is giving medication-assisted treatment (such as methadone) to an IV drug user who presents with a complicated abscess and cellulitis. Negotiating the palliation of withdrawal as part of the admission may even reduce future risk of serious infection by helping her not engage in injection drug use.

An openly discussed risk assessment that uses common language and readily understandable statistics is helpful and necessary but not sufficient when managing a case where the patient disagrees with treatment. Making a choice to receive adequate care by meeting a patient halfway is better than providing statistics or documenting conversations. This is especially relevant with a permissive discharge. An example of a permissive discharge familiar to most emergency physicians is the individual with low-risk chest pain who has unaddressed risk factors. A physician's recommendation about admission or discharge may rely on gestalt in these situations, and a reasonable patient's objection to admission could adjust the physician's plan. This is especially pertinent if a viable plan to continue evaluation and treatment as an outpatient is put into place. Practically, the difference between a persuasive discharge and a permissive one is that the outcome lands closer to the physician's ideal with a persuasive approach, while the permissive approach settles more closely with the patient's wishes. Both provide acceptable alternatives, especially in comparison to an AMA discharge situation in which the patient does not accept any further treatment.

No matter the disposition decision, exploring motivations for the patient's decision is necessary. Is he scared of the diagnosis or the treatment? Is there a situation at home that is distracting her from the decision? Is he considering short-term and long-term consequences of the decision? The particular components of the conversation make a better record of the conversation and the patient's motivations than a fill-in-the-blank form [1]. Conversely, using an AMA form, and by extension the "AMA" moniker, has the frequent effect of being manipulative. The myths and surrounding AMA discharges described above should be avoided when motivating patients to complete treatment in the ED. Using myths, stereotypes, and a complicated form can each undermine the patient-provider relationship and can harm the chances of the patient seeking the best outcome, either in this visit or as part of follow-up.

The paternalistic approach to AMA discharge is separate from strategies that use negotiation and motivation. It should only be used in cases where the patient lacks capacity to make health decisions and no surrogate is easily or readily available. This occurs more frequently in the ED than most other contexts. Intoxication and unstable mental illness are the most frequent reasons why a patient should be denied an AMA discharge. Nonetheless, thorough documentation of the patient's motivations, as well as results from an assessment of capacity (also documented), should be made [18]. Psychiatric history and specific delusional or other psychotic behaviors should be noted. In many instances, lack of capacity from intoxication may benefit from objective data (e.g., blood alcohol levels) supporting it. The test of clinical sobriety often applied in the ED to decide about appropriate discharge does not rely on alcohol levels and can be sufficient when deciding when to release an intoxicated patient, but the objectivity of impaired capacity for the purposes of AMA discharge is strengthened with the serum or breath alcohol level. Ethicists and medical providers have lessened the use of the terminology of paternalism in medical practice, but in the instance of incapacitation, denying an AMA discharge is the ethical choice for the patient's care. Until capacity is restored or a surrogate is identified, the incapacitated patient with urgent medical need should not be discharged, and accompanying chemical or physical restraint to prevent harm to self or staff may be indicated.

A signed AMA form to release a patient AMA is not a substitute for an informed consent discussion and may stigmatize the encounter. Any discharge approach should attempt to minimize harm to the individual by recommending care within the identified constraints set by the patient. This includes providing medical treatment before release, appropriate prescriptions, and arranged follow-up. An open invitation to return to the ED for continued treatment should be maintained by the provider and by the individual, who is often the nurse, discharging the patient. Maintaining access to care and keeping open the possibility for a treatment plan promotes the patient's health and their right to self-determination.

Case Conclusions and Analysis

Case 1: Precious

This case of a patient with an emergent potentially life-threatening condition (i.e., acute appendicitis) illustrates the context in which many ED patients interact with health care. Mr. Strong's stated priority is the care of his dog. Absent the ability to provide direct care for the pet, and in the context of clear capacity, he wants to delay treatment until he can assure the dog's well-being. Although this deals with pets, this situation can be transposed onto patient obligations to family members, jobs, and others. Understanding the patient's motivations may provide information that will help the provider to persuade the patient to receive care for his appendicitis. If creative solutions including social work intervention or the care team calling family or neighbors cannot keep him in the hospital, *persuading* the patient with decision-making capacity to return as soon as he is able while *permitting* him to carry out his personal business is the ethically justifiable, preferable option. Approaches to reduce risk include treatment with outpatient oral, broad-spectrum antibiotics for abdominal pathogens [19, 20] followed by persistent callbacks to check in with him. Analgesia should not be withheld so as not to violate the ethical principle of nonmaleficence. This permissive approach, when the patient's rightful authority is highlighted, can make it easier for the patient to agree to stay. Any efforts to persuade him to stay in the hospital should be documented, as should the provider's judgment of Mr. Strong's capacity. If adequate documentation is made, a specific AMA form need not be completed but could aid in directing the conversation with the patient about the risks of discharge. If he leaves, this would be a *permissive* AMA discharge.

Case 2: Smoke 'Em if You Got 'Em

Cases with medical issues similar to Ms. Do's are becoming more common, especially given the expanded legalization of medical and recreational marijuana. Her case represents two common types of potentially frustrating patient encounters in the ED: first is the patient seeking opiate pain medications with a clear medical indication, and second is the patient who will not accept a diagnosis. The risk in this case includes an unidentified secondary diagnosis, patient elopement (LWBD), and litigation in the case of a bad outcome. However it forms, poor rapport between patient and physician is a barrier to optimal care and increases the likelihood of legal action, independent of an AMA discharge outcome. By intentionally suspending judgment of the patient's decisions and building rapport by treating her decisions as being within her right, the provider may reduce the likelihood of the patient LWBD or leaving AMA. Independent of individual or institutional policies about opiate analgesia, offering IV fluids and antiemetics as well as a nicotine patch may palliate her symptoms and express provider concern while a medical workup is ongoing. Considering alternative treatments (such as IV haloperidol) for cyclic vomiting, abdominal migraines, or marijuana hyperemesis syndrome may yield a medical outcome that mitigates the risk of this encounter and improves the patient-provider rapport. Expressing empathy in the form of an apology or other bridge to common ground respects the patient's autonomy and supports beneficent clinical decisions. These approaches represent the *persuasive* approach that can prevent AMA discharge.

Case 3: "Come on Guys!"

Transient incapacitation from substance use disorders is a common challenge to patient's decision-making in the emergency department; it is so common that emergency providers often overlook intoxication as an ethical issue. Despite his partial insight into his alcohol dependence, Hector does not have full decisional capacity. We do not know if he is intoxicated, withdrawing, or both; he also has the potential for life-threatening intracranial injury and is exhibiting behavior just outside his baseline disagreeable (but not typically aggressive) personality. If granted his stated wishes, he would be released, perhaps with unidentified injuries or illnesses, and might seek additional alcohol. Paying careful attention to his agitation provides ethical support for a decision to physically or chemically restrain him in order to prevent harm. By simultaneously sedating and treating possible alcohol withdrawal, benzodiazepines provide a strategy to minimize risk of harm to the patient or the ED staff. Documenting decision-making capacity or lack thereof, attempting to identify and contact an authorized surrogate decision-maker, and using time stamps or serum alcohol levels will support a decision to act in the patient's interest while he is intoxicated. Capacity is not entirely dependent on intoxication levels, however. If a CT of the head and a trauma survey reveal no acute injury, the most likely diagnosis is alcohol withdrawal. The appropriately paternalistic decision to rule out threatening injuries may shift to a more permissive approach of discharge that confers respect for autonomy and enables future encounters.

Final Thoughts

Neither patients nor emergency providers prefer to be involved in an AMA discharge. An intentional process to reduce negative outcomes from patients leaving before treatment completion can improve patient outcomes and reduce liability and could even reduce the frequency of AMA cases. Whether it is the AIMED method or an approach as we suggest that implements a persuasive, permissive, or paternalistic strategy to negotiate optimal care, AMA discharges should be safe and rare and promote harm reduction. Institutional guidelines should favor meaningful documentation of the encounter that cites decisional capacity, patient understanding of consequences, and a reasonable alternative plan for treatment over boilerplate legal documents. A compassionate approach to patient care, even when the patient's preference contrasts with the provider's recommendations, can satisfy the patient's right of autonomy and physician's aspiration to provide the best care even within an AMA discharge situation.

Acknowledgments With acknowledgment to Rishana Cohen, MD, and Michal Poplawski, MD.

References

1. Clark MA, Abbott JT, Adyanthaya T. Ethics seminars: a best-practice approach to navigating the against-medical-advice discharge. Acad Emerg Med. 2014;21(9):1050–7.
2. Ibrahim SA, Kwoh CK, Krishnan E. Factors associated with patients who leave acute-care hospitals against medical advice. Am J Public Health. 2007;12(97):2204–8.
3. Jerrard DA, Chasm RM. Patients leaving against medical advice (AMA) from the emergency department – disease prevalence and willingness to return. J Emerg Med. 2009;41(4):412–7.
4. Pham JC, Ho GK, Hill PM, McCarthy ML, Pronovost PJ. National study of patient, visit, and hospital characteristics associated with leaving an emergency department without being seen: predicting LWBS. Acad Emerg Med. 2009;16(10):949–55.
5. Polevoi SK, Quinn JV, Kramer NR. Factors associated with patients who leave without being seen. Acad Emerg Med. 2005;12(3):232–6.

6. Reinke DA, Walker M, Boslaugh S, Hodge D. Predictors of pediatric emergency patients discharged against medical advice. Clin Pediatr. 2009;48(3):263–70.
7. Sun BC, Binstadt ES, Pelletier A, Camargo CA. Characteristics and temporal trends of "left without being seen" visits in US emergency departments, 1995–2002. J Emerg Med. 2006;32(2):211–5.
8. Tothy AS, Staley S, Dean EK, Johnson S, Johnson D. Pediatric left-without-being-seen patients: what happens to them after they leave the pediatric emergency department? Pediatr Emerg Care. 2013;29(11):1194–6.
9. Wilson BJ, Zimmerman D, Applebaum KG, Kovalski N, Stein C. Patients who leave before being seen in an urgent care setting. Eur J Emerg Med. 2013;20(6):420–4.
10. Wigder HN, Leslie K, Mathew A. Insurance companies refusing payment for patients who leave the emergency department against medical advice is a myth. Ann Emerg Med. 2010;55(4):393.
11. Levy F, Mareiniss DP, Iacovelli C. The importance of a proper against-medical-advice (AMA) discharge: how signing out AMA may create significant liability protection for providers. J Emerg Med. 2010;43(3):516–20.
12. Stearns CR, Bakamijan A, Sattar S, Ritterman Weintraub M. Discharges against medical advice at a county hospital: provider perceptions and practice. J Hosp Med. 2017;12(1):11–7.
13. Sullivan W. Special report: AMA discharges. ED Leg Lett. 2007;18(6):66–8.
14. Welsh S, Kauer K, Fontenot SF. Risk management and the emergency department. ACEP; 2011. http://www.acep.org/News-Media-top-banner/EMTALA. Accessed Feb 2017.
15. EMTALA Q & A. Emergency Department Management. 2003. https://www.ahcmedia.com/articles/print/22468-emtala-q-a.
16. Brenner J, Joslin J, Goulette A, Wojcik S, Grant W. Against medical advice: a survey of ED clinicians' rationale for use. J Emerg Nurs. 2016;42(5):408–11.
17. Furukawa MF. Electronic medical records and the efficiency of hospital emergency departments. Med Care Res Rev. 2011;68(1):75–95.
18. Appelbaum PS. Assessment of patients' competence to consent to treatment. N Engl J Med. 2007;357:1834–40.
19. Hansson J, Körner U, Ludwigs K, Johnsson E, Jönsson C, Lundholm K. Antibiotics as first-line therapy for acute appendicitis: evidence for a change in clinical practice. World J Surg. 2012;36(9):2028–36.
20. Salminen P, Paajanen H, Rautio T, Nordström P, Aarnio M, Rantanen T, et al. Antibiotic therapy vs appendectomy for treatment of uncomplicated acute appendicitis: the APPAC randomized clinical trial. JAMA. 2015;313(23):2340–8.

Chapter 9
To Thy Own Self Be True: Contributions from Consultation-Liaison Psychiatry

Nicole Allen and Philip R. Muskin

Introduction

The decision by a patient to leave the hospital against medical advice has many psychiatric elements. Not only are psychiatric comorbidities common among patients who request to leave the hospital against medical advice (AMA), but the decision by a patient to leave an acute medical hospitalization AMA is usually prompted by a desperate belief, often rooted in fear or anger, that there are no other options. The literature on psychiatric elements in AMA discharges began with two psychoanalytically trained consultation-liaison psychiatrists who found that understanding the patient's motivation requesting to leave AMA is important [1]. Their findings remain current today. On discharge over half of a population of patients who left the hospital AMA were found to be anxious or agitated [2], and the majority of patients who reach the decision to leave AMA would choose to resolve the issues prompting their request if given the option [1].

This chapter will consider patient requests to leave AMA from a psychodynamic perspective and will discuss requests to leave AMA during a medical hospitalization in patients with psychiatric comorbidities. The first section of this chapter presents case examples of patients requesting discharge against medical advice and typical physician reactions. The second section discusses comorbid psychiatric disorders and requests for discharge AMA. The final section discusses the role of the psychiatric consultant in evaluating patients who request to leave the hospital AMA.

N. Allen
Department of Psychiatry, Lenox Hill Hospital, New York, NY, USA

P. R. Muskin (✉)
Consultation-Liaison Psychiatry, Columbia University Medical Center, New York, NY, USA
e-mail: prm1@cumc.columbia.edu

© Springer International Publishing AG, part of Springer Nature 2018
D. Alfandre (ed.), *Against-Medical-Advice Discharges from the Hospital*,
https://doi.org/10.1007/978-3-319-75130-6_9

Transference and Countertransference

Patients requesting to leave AMA can provoke a variety of reactions from their treatment team. The physician may like the patient immensely and want the patient to stay in the hospital and continue treatment, making an enormous effort to convince the patient to remain admitted. Conversely, the physician may intensely hate the patient and feel relieved that he wants to sign out AMA and offer little resistance to the patient's plan of action. There is nothing inherently wrong or preventable regarding an emotional reaction to a patient; every physician will have certain types of patients she/he finds charming or irritating, while certain patients will elicit unavoidable reactions in their physicians due to some aspect of the patient's personality or behavior. What is important is recognizing and understanding thoughts or feelings on the part of the physician that may interfere with objective, equitable treatment of all patients.

Differentiating reactions to patients that stem from something the patient provokes versus reactions that stem from the physician's personal experiences is an important mental exercise that promotes better care. Some patients provoke the same reaction in most physicians; however, their personal experiences and relationships create a susceptibility to experiencing a certain type of patient in a unique individualized manner. For example, a patient who is loud and aggressive, not trusting his doctors because he sees the world as hostile and is trying to not feel vulnerable, elicits fear and avoidance in many of his physicians. The physician's response to this patient's affect and behavior is countertransference or a reaction to a patient that is largely instigated by the patient's behavior. On the other hand, a physician who angrily feels that his father withheld approval of him may be susceptible to experience an elderly male patient as judging his abilities as a medical provider with little other evidence supporting this assumption. The physician relates negatively to his patient with little from the patient to provoke the reaction; this is transference. Transference is a redirection of unconscious feelings and tendencies, usually originating in childhood, from one person to another. In the first case, the physician is having an understandable reaction to a patient's behavior that is likely shared by many staff members interacting with that patient. In the second case, it may be appropriate for the physician to seek out peer supervision or his or her own personal therapy to explore why certain patients elicit a response not experienced by the majority of staff members and to find ways to manage the response when it happens.

These concepts remind physicians that it is vital to be aware of their own emotional reactions that may interfere with rational consideration of patients' requests to leave AMA, whether global or particular to a certain physician-patient interaction. Below are some case examples designed to demonstrate common emotional reactions to different patient presentations.

Anger

A 68-year-old man with a history of alcohol use disorder is admitted for treatment of alcohol withdrawal. He has been admitted four times in the past 3 months. He is homeless, and it appears he presents to the hospital when he runs out of money. He has a history of alcohol withdrawal seizures and has required admission to the ICU for treatment of alcohol withdrawal in the past. On interview you find him loud, rude, and unpleasant. He refuses an addiction psychiatry consult and says his drinking is not a problem. On day 2 of his admission, he demands to speak to the floor social worker regarding housing and obtaining benefits. He becomes agitated and threatening toward staff when the social worker does not come to see him quickly enough. He demands to leave the hospital despite the high doses of benzo-diazepines he currently requires to treat his withdrawal.

Most physicians who have spent time working in an emergency room or in an inpatient unit will have encountered at least one patient with a substance use disorder (frequently alcohol use disorder) who repeatedly presents for treatment of withdrawal. The treating physician, in an attempt to interrupt the cycle of intoxication and withdrawal, may emphatically encourage the patient to be treated in a rehab facility or agree to outpatient substance use treatment; although rates of alcohol use treatment acceptance may be higher than physicians expect (66% to almost 100% in a 2011 Danish population) [3], substance use interventions may still be rejected by the patient. The patient may have tried this treatment in the past with little success, or the patient may be in denial regarding the impact of alcohol on his health and social situation. Rejection of the appropriate treatment can understandably lead the physician to feel helpless and exploited. The physician may think, "This patient is just going to go back out and drink again and then come back to the hospital." He may be conflicted in wanting to release the patient and subconsciously hoping the patient will have a withdrawal seizure as punishment while also worrying that the patient will have a bad outcome and the doctor will be blamed. Hearing that there is a patient with a long history of alcohol use disorder and frequent admissions for treatment of alcohol withdrawal can lead to some of these thoughts arising before even meeting the patient.

When confronted with a patient who generally interacts with others in an aggressive, entitled manner, the understandable immediate reaction of the physician is anger and withdrawal. Although interactions with this patient are likely rarely pleasant, considering some of the motivations behind the patient's behavior might be useful in helping the physician feel less frustrated and exploited. While outside the hospital, this homeless patient is likely in an environment in which showing any sign of weakness is dangerous; in order to avoid being victimized, he has learned to present a loud, aggressive front. He does this in every situation regardless of the environment. Although his actions are often maladaptive when he is not on the streets, he has learned that there are times when being loud and aggressive get him what he wants more quickly. From this perspective, his behavior could be considered resourceful. Trying to help the patient understand that his behavior works in reverse while hospitalized, while acknowledging that it is vital on the street, may enable the physician to prevent a crisis between the patient and staff resulting in his request to sign out.

Thus an understanding of the etiology of this patient's behavior might be helpful to the physician; however, this does not mean that the behavior should go unchallenged. Although attempting to maintain an alliance with the patient will aid in productive treatment, tolerating assaultive behavior or threats of physical violence does not benefit the patient or the staff. The patient should be informed that yelling and threats are not tolerated and will result in security presence in order to maintain patient and staff safety. At times the presence of a uniformed security officer, even if outside of the patient's room, has the effect of "we mean business." The physician should speak in a calm but assertive voice and avoid matching the patient in volume of speech or aggressive demeanor, which will frequently instigate further agitation from the patient. Patients often respond favorably to the phrase "I can't hear what you're saying when you yell." Reminding the patient that we are here to help him and that he deserves to be helped can be validating to the patient (using the word "deserves" speaks to the patient's needs). At the same time, we need to be clear that we cannot give him what he deserves if he scares everyone or acts in a manner that is threatening. While it may be a cliché, most everyone understands the meaning of, "you can catch more flies with honey than with vinegar." When this patient is requesting discharge against medical advice, the physician should consider the reasons the patient might be requesting discharge, the potential dangers of allowing the patient to leave the hospital, and any emotions or attitudes that might cloud the physician's objective evaluation regarding the dangers of the patient leaving the hospital. In the case above, the patient is at risk for withdrawal seizures and possibly death, and a request to leave AMA may prompt a psychiatric evaluation for capacity.

Sadness

A 49-year-old woman with metastatic cervical cancer is admitted to the hospital for failure to thrive. She has been admitted three times in the last few months for the same reason. Because of her limited life expectancy, in each admission she is encouraged to discuss inpatient hospice; however, the patient consistently declines and signs herself out. She is divorced, has two children who are not very close to her, and neither her children nor other relatives have visited her in the hospital. She believes her cancer diagnosis is unfair and wonders if she is being punished for her poor relationships with her children. She is calm and cooperative but is reluctant to engage in a goals-of-care discussion. She cries frequently. She will not discuss hospice and eventually requests to go home and manage her affairs alone.

Although the first reaction of the treating physician to this patient might be annoyance that she is interfering with expedient and medically appropriate transfer to hospice, this most likely masks an underlying corresponding sense of despair and helplessness. This patient's prognosis is poor, treatment has been ineffective, and she is lamenting that she will end her life with poor relationships with her loved ones. Patients such as this one may elicit powerful feelings of sadness given we all have some fear of dying alone and are dissatisfied with life.

Most patients react with sadness when presented with news of a terminal illness or potentially life-threatening diagnosis. Common reactions include (but are not limited to) shock, questioning, and tearfulness. Some degrees of sadness or grief are appropriate reactions to receiving news of a terminal illness; however, acute depression is not a maladaptive response to bad news but a psychiatric illness requiring evaluation and treatment. Depression, unlike typical sadness, is characterized by guilt, self-loathing, and self-recrimination [4]. The depressed patient may blame herself for her illness and may not participate in recommended medical care. She may feel that she has lost her identity now that she is ill. Patients who are depressed and hopeless regarding their medical diagnosis can evoke similar feelings in the treating physician. In this case the physician must be careful to continue reviewing and developing the plan of care actively as opposed to aligning with the patient's sense of hopelessness and lethargy. Conversely putting pressure on the patient to consent to hospice may feel to her like the physician is not listening to her concerns. The patient may benefit from assistance reaching out to her children. She may have financial issues pending at home she feels she must attend to and could benefit from social work involvement. She may believe hospice to be a facility where patients go to suffer and die alone. She could benefit from a palliative care consult to more fully understand what hospice entails. If interventions such as these fail and the patient still insists on leaving AMA despite her clear inability to care for herself at home alone, it may be helpful to call a psychiatry consult to assist with appropriate treatment of the patient's depression.

Guilt

A previously healthy 65-year-old man is admitted to the hospital for worsening weakness and poor appetite. He is found to have a pancreatic pseudocyst. It is determined that no intervention is needed for the pseudocyst, and this is likely not the cause of his anorexia. A psychiatry consult is called to assess for depression, and the consultant does not find the patient to have a major depressive disorder. The lack of a clear etiology for the patient's symptoms is frustrating for both patient and physician. Soon after admission the patient develops a C. difficile infection. He continues to become weaker and anorexic and loses more weight. Prior to admission he was active and lived independently. He has many friends but only allows his cousin to visit him because he doesn't want anyone to see him in his current debilitated state. After over a month in the hospital with no improvement, the medical team recommends continued inpatient evaluation and treatment. He requests to go home with his brother.

The majority of medical education is focused on treating the patient effectively. When this doesn't happen, e.g., the patient's cancer progresses, his heart failure worsens while he waits for a heart transplant, or his deficits following stroke are worse than expected, the physician can feel powerless and guilty. As opposed to the case of the depressed terminally ill patient, this situation may lead to patient and physician frustration and demoralization. When the patient gives up and requests to leave, the physician may readily agree because she/he feels like a failure. Some physicians may subconsciously blame the patient himself for failing treatment. This creates a difficult dynamic of blame and guilt between the patient and the physician [5]. There is no clear solution to this type of case that satisfies all involved; it may be appropriate to arrange for discharge to a nursing facility with no discrete diagnosis identified. In any case, the physician should be open with the patient about his or her lack of insight into the patient's symptoms and allow the patient to express his frustration.

Overidentification

A 21-year-old woman with a history of alcohol use disorder is admitted for acute pancreatitis. This is her first admission related to her alcohol use. She is a college student at a prestigious university where she has a high GPA and participates in multiple extracurricular activities. She intends to apply to medical school after a gap year of volunteering in Ghana. She has an engaging personality, a winning sense of humor, and is well liked by the medical team. She is successfully treated for her pancreatitis, and the team has recommended transfer for inpatient alcohol addiction treatment. The patient cooperates with a psychiatry consult and initially is considering transfer to an inpatient unit; however, she is ambivalent regarding treatment. The physician has several lengthy conversations with her about the benefits of treating her alcohol use disorder and the potential danger if she continues drinking at her current intake level. Initially she agrees to treatment only if she is transferred to a particular private facility that she and her family are unable to afford. When offered multiple alternative options that are equally acceptable, and in similar locations, she declines the referrals and requests to sign out of the hospital.

This patient, though presenting with an alcohol use disorder, is different in many respects from the patient presented in the first case. Young physicians could feel they have much in common with a bright college student intending to apply to medical school, and older physicians may see in her a chance to rectify past personal errors. We are all vulnerable to identify with our patients in a variety of ways. Some patients are very much like us in age, appearance, background, professional goals, and so on. Some patients remind us of ourselves, even if we are not consciously aware of the experience. The more "like us" someone is, the more the probability that our response to the patient may be influenced by those feelings. Had the patient in the "Anger" example been successfully treated and refused rehabilitation, he likely would be discharged immediately. This patient may elicit a physician's desire to go above and beyond in terms of pressure to submit to the recommendation for inpatient addiction treatment. The team might agonize over "letting" her sign out when in reality this patient, although potentially making a choice that doesn't prioritize her health, is medically ready for discharge and does not need to sign out "against medical advice." Although she would clearly benefit from substance use treatment, she is not currently in the necessary state of mind to engage in appropriate treatment.

The patient clearly presents an element of willful sabotage of the referral process. She expresses a desire to get treatment for a serious and life-threatening addiction but makes it impossible to send her by requiring a unique and unreasonable facility. At the same time, she engages the treatment team in a frustrating back and forth that is ultimately fruitless. It might be difficult for the team to recognize her actions for what they are given her otherwise pleasant and engaging demeanor, but ultimately, this patient should be offered substance use treatment referrals and discharged.

Apathy

A 35-year-old man with a history of intravenous (IV) heroin use is admitted for the second time with bacterial endocarditis requiring several weeks of IV antibiotics. He is unable to be transferred to a nursing facility to complete his course of antibiotics due to lack of insurance. Thus he will need to stay in the hospital for another 6 weeks. The primary team is fearful that he will use his IV access to use heroin if discharged with a PICC line. He professes that he wants to quit drugs forever; however, this is one of the many times that he has made the same statement and he has continued to use heroin. He is vocally appreciative of the care he is receiving in the hospital and proclaims during every interaction, "you're the best doctors I've ever had!" Initially he says he is willing to remain in the hospital for his entire course of antibiotics because he wants to "get better." Ten days later he states that he misses his family who live too far away to visit him. Physically he appears much better than he did upon admission and has no other acute medical issues. Eventually, with little resistance from the treatment team, he says that he wants to check himself out of the hospital and discontinue the IV treatment.

This patient, similar to the first case presented in this chapter, has a relapsing substance use disorder that has directly caused several hospital admissions. He creates feelings of powerlessness and sometimes a desire to avoid the patient on the part of the physician: powerlessness due to his history of relapsing substance use and avoidance due to his loud but somewhat artificial proclamations of appreciation for his treatment and intentions to stay sober. The latter statements are an expression of the patient's own desperate hope that this admission will result in a different outcome for him; unlike the first patient, he seems aware of the general desirability of sobriety but feels somewhat doubtful underneath his surface enthusiasm that he will be able to quit his use of heroin.

Because of these feelings of helplessness and distaste, and the patient's ostensible physical improvement and lack of successful drug rehabilitation in the past, his physician may feel that he has done all he can for the patient and do little to try to convince the patient to remain in the hospital. In contrast to the young college student, the team might feel a sense of relief and feel the urge to immediately acquiesce to the patient's request. Although the patient may eventually come to the same conclusions about prioritizing family matters over his own medical treatment, he still merits an in-depth discussion of the risks of leaving the hospital prior to release.

Psychiatric Comorbidities and Leaving AMA

Studies consistently show that patients who leave the hospital AMA have higher rates of psychiatric illness and substance use disorders [6–9]. In general, medical hospitalizations are stressful, and patients with psychiatric disorders may be less able to handle stress adaptively. This can interfere with collaborative discharge planning [10]. Medical hospitalizations raise clear issues such as financial stress, absence from work and activities, separation from friends and family, boredom, pain and other physical discomforts, lack of sleep, and worry over outcome. Being hospitalized stimulates psychodynamic issues of dependence, loss of control, and fears of one's mortality. Certain patients may react to hospitalizations with maladaptive regression, becoming unnecessarily dependent on nurses and other care providers for feeding, changing, and ambulation. Some patients may feel threatened by the lack of control over their health and react by constantly challenging the medical team. Others feel a great sense of distress, whether merited or not, that they might die during their admission. Although anyone could experience these emotions in times of stress, these reactions can be exaggerated in patients with psychotic, mood, or personality disorders and lead to maladaptive behaviors.

The following sections will discuss the relationship between specific psychiatric diagnoses and requests to leave AMA along with suggested approaches to these patients in a medical setting.

Substance Use

Substance misuse is a significant predictor of requests to leave the hospital AMA [11–15]. In one study, 83.5% of patients admitted to the hospital in an area of northern Italy with clinical conditions related to substance use or substance use disorders were discharged AMA [8]. Among patients who leave the hospital AMA, those with alcohol abuse are much more likely to re-present to the hospital within 15 days [16].

Assessing and ameliorating common causes of AMA requests from patients with substance use disorders can help prevent early discharges. Doctors and nurses often perceive patients with substance use disorders negatively as "drug seekers"; patients are sensitive to this bias and often react with anger toward their treatment team [1]. Physicians should approach every patient with a calm, unprejudiced attitude [15]. The physician should assess for withdrawal and cravings and use the appropriate psychopharmacological treatment to help keep patients comfortable, potentially with the assistance of an addiction psychiatrist or general consultation-liaison psychiatrist when available. Patients in alcohol withdrawal should be appropriately assessed using the CIWA-Ar scale and adequately treated using PO or IV benzodiazepines [17]. For patients with opiate use disorders and acute medical issues, the priority should not be immediately weaned off opiate pain medications. Patients with opiate dependence should be adequately treated for pain, and patients already on methadone maintenance treatment should be continued on methadone while admitted with additional pain medication administered if indicated. In some cases, inducing the patient with buprenorphine and appropriate follow-up with an outpatient treatment center will be of tremendous value.

Many physicians feel the responsibility to reform patients with substance use disorders by detoxing them in the hospital or referring them to addiction-centered outpatient treatments upon discharge. Physicians and other staff may experience negative feelings toward these patients as they present repeatedly to the hospital for treatment of the same symptoms (e.g., withdrawal in the patient with alcohol use disorder or chest pain in the patient with cocaine use disorder), which are perceived as self-induced. Although it is appropriate to offer a patient with a substance use disorder treatment in the form of inpatient rehabilitation, inpatient detox, or outpatient services such as medication-assisted treatment (e.g., methadone maintenance, buprenorphine), it is important for the physician to appreciate the "stage of change" of each patient. This will avoid significant frustration on the part of the patient and the physician [18]. Patients who are in the "pre-contemplation" stage are unaware of the severity of their substance use issues and will be unreceptive to attempts to facilitate treatment. Patients in the "contemplation" stage are aware of their problems and may be receptive to intervention but have not yet made a commitment to take action. Patients in the "preparation" stage are ready to take action to address their substance issues within the next month, and patients in the "action" stage are in the midst of treatment. During the "maintenance" stage, patients are working to prevent relapse. Although always appropriate to present patients with the services that are available to treat substance use issues, pressuring patients who are in the pre-contemplation stage is rarely useful. Motivational interviewing is an approach that takes the patient where he or she is and works toward taking responsibility for making changes [19].

Psychotic Disorders

Patients with psychotic disorders such as schizophrenia who are admitted to the hospital for medical conditions can present in a variety of ways. Many patients have a long history of mental health treatment, and their symptoms are well controlled. Others may have not been in mental health treatment for some time and are actively symptomatic. Of those who are currently symptomatic, some may be clearly psychotic with delusional thinking or auditory hallucinations, while others may be more subtly paranoid and irritable.

Although psychosis or schizophrenia can interfere with decision-making from both emotional and neurocognitive perspectives [20], it is important to be aware that patients who have active psychotic disorders may still have the capacity to make medical decisions including to participate in discharge planning. It is only when the psychotic disorder interferes with the patient's ability to rationally manipulate the information that the illness itself results in a lack of capacity to make decisions. Patients who report currently experiencing auditory hallucinations or "hearing voices" may still be able to understand their medical situation and appreciate the consequences of their decision, while patients who are quietly irritable and delusional may appear to understand their medical conditions and course but upon more thorough interview are making medical decisions about their own care in an irrational manner.

As in the general patient population, education and counseling can improve the ability of patients with schizophrenia to make their medical decisions [20]. When a patient who is psychotic requests to leave, physicians should attempt to clearly explain the indication for continued hospital admission and address any irrational ideas the patient may have regarding his medical care. A psychiatry consult should be called if there is uncertainty about whether or not the patient's mental illness is interfering with their ability to make medical decisions and if psychiatric treatment can help. At times, treatment over objection, even on a medical/surgical service, will restore the patient's capacity to make informed decisions. If the psychosis interferes with the patient's ability to make a decision regarding urgent medical care, treatment with an antipsychotic medication is an important step in restoring the patient's capacity.

Mood Disorders

Mood disorders are among the top five primary admission diagnoses of people who leave the hospital against medical advice [14]. Patients may present as either depressed, with low mood and neurovegetative symptoms, or manic, with elevated or irritable affect and pressured speech.

Patients who appear depressed may have a preexisting major depressive disorder or may have a sad reaction to a medical hospitalization. Distinguishing sadness from a clinical depression is possible based on expert evaluation. Sadness is a normal reaction to bad news with little other emotional or cognitive effects. Patients who are depressed are more likely to cognitively distort facts about their illness, treatment course, and prognosis in a negativistic manner leading to a pessimistic view of outcome [20]. This may prompt requests to leave the hospital AMA. Some physicians may be quick to assume patients who are tearful in reaction to bad news are "depressed," while others may assume that depression is a normal response to medical illness and miss the opportunity to appropriately treat a major depression. When a depressed patient requests discharge AMA, gentle exploration to assess for potential skewing of judgment is appropriate. Physicians should be careful not to mirror the patient's negativism and to actively urge the patient to select appropriately aggressive treatment for both his medical condition and his depression.

It is important to be aware of the patient who requests discharge AMA in order to die. The motivation of the patient to request discharge in this case should be carefully explored. This request may not necessarily be due to depression although this should be considered. A patient may request death due to untreated pain, a need for control over his illness, or feelings of rage or guilt [5]. No request to die should ever go unexplored. The discussion between patient and physician has the potential for a profound interaction. Automatic "yes" or "no" does not permit the discovery of the powerful emotions that fuel the patient's request nor does it allow the physician to self-reflect on what "yes" or "no" means. As more states continue to approve physician-assisted death, the physician will ultimately lose the opportunity to hastily end the discussion with the statement "it is not legal in our state."

There is little data available on patients in the midst of an acute manic episode and AMA discharges from medical admissions. In general, patients who are acutely manic and request to leave the hospital AMA are unlikely to be able to rationally prioritize their health over outside tasks of perceived importance. A psychiatry consult should be called to evaluate patients who are euphoric or irritable, not sleeping, and uninterruptible when speaking, all suggestive of acute mania, especially if requesting to leave the hospital AMA.

Personality Disorders

Patients with personality disorders are among the most difficult patients to treat in the hospital. Typically, they have poor internal strategies for coping with stress and are more likely to resort to immature mechanisms to mitigate their anxieties. Many clinicians will find these behaviors challenging to address [21]. We will focus on the three personality disorders that pose the highest probability of the patient signing out AMA.

Patients with borderline personality disorder may "split" the hospital staff. They construct the world as "good" or "bad." Secondary to their personality structure, they are incapable of perceiving both "good" and "bad" characteristics within the same person at the same time. This defense mechanism results in the patient experiencing some staff at certain times as all "good" and others as all "bad." Thus the patient relates to some staff with what seems to be a close connection while vilifying other staff members. These "relationships" may turn 180 degrees in an instant, confusing and angering those suddenly on the "bad" side of the split. The patient with borderline personality disorder is at risk for making impulsive, nonproductive decisions such as signing out AMA in reaction to a perceived interpersonal slight. Such patients can be extremely sensitive to rejection and may interpret the most benign remark as a sign that the physician has decided she/he is unlovable or undeserving. Although these patients often would be assessed as having the capacity to make these decisions, the rationale for their choices to terminate medical care often appears to be trivial.

Once a borderline patient feels slighted and subsequently emotionally vulnerable and decides to leave AMA, rational discussion may have little impact. In order to best avoid this scenario, when treating a patient with borderline personality disorder, it is important to set clear expectations with boundaries from the beginning in terms of intimacy (e.g., sharing personal information) and attention (i.e., spending appropriate but limited amounts of time with the patient throughout the day).

The patient with paranoid personality disorder is suspicious of others without meeting criteria for schizophrenia (i.e., without delusions or hallucinations). This patient may be quick to believe that others, including his physicians, have caused or are contributing to his illness [22]. It is essential to keep the paranoid patient aware of the medical plan as quickly and clearly as possible in order to as best as possible prevent him from believing information is being kept from him and attempting to sign out AMA.

The narcissistic patient feels superior to others. Illness causes a perception of threats to his own self-image of perfection. In order to counteract these feelings, these patients act as if they are superior to everyone else. The patient may insist that the most senior physician on the staff take care of him, belittling house staff as "inadequate." When staff attempt to verify the patient's claims by looking the patient up on the Internet, they may find nothing to support the patient's perceived VIP status. This may result in a physician's skepticism of the patient's claims and a likely unproductive confrontation of the patient's demeaning behavior. When the patient threatens to call his "friends in high places" to complain, the reality is that such "friends" are well aware of the patient's behavior and are extremely understanding of the burden of caring for him. Caring for the narcissistic patient can be particularly frustrating as confrontation is likely to result in the patient signing out AMA in spite of the medical risks. The medical risks may seem inconsequential to the patient compared to the psychological "insult." Although it may be irksome, the most effective way to calm the narcissistic patient is to not indulge the patient's need to be superior without belittling the patient. When angered at the unavoidable inconveniences or delays that occur during hospitalizations, the physician can calm the patient down by asking for his indulgence to "rise above" such occurrences.

Role of the Psychiatric Consultant in Discharges Against Medical Advice

Psychiatric consultants are most commonly included in the care of a patient who requests to leave the hospital AMA in order to determine whether the patient has decision-making capacity to make that decision. Many physicians erroneously believe they are obligated to request a psychiatric consult for capacity evaluations; however, any physician may make a capacity evaluation. For instance, when there is a decision to be made relating to the care of a patient with advanced dementia or a patient who is sedated and intubated in the intensive care unit, it is usually quite clear that the patient does not have capacity to make his own decisions. On the other hand, a 1989 study showed that patients with a psychiatry consult early in the admission were more likely to choose to remain hospitalized [10].

The request for a psychiatric consultation regarding a patient's capacity is where the emotions of the requesting physician may influence an unrecognized "wish" to believe that the patient has capacity to sign out. Kornfeld et al. [23] found an 80% concordance rate (41/51) when the psychiatric consultant agreed with the determination by the primary team of the patient's lack of capacity to make medical decisions. When the primary team assessed the patient to have capacity, the psychiatric consultant agreed only 37.5% (9/24) of the time. This decreased concordance rate in patients thought to have capacity by the referring physician was corroborated by another 2009 study [24]. In the nonconcordant group (where the referring physicians believed the patients to have capacity), almost half were threatening to leave AMA. In the nonconcordant group (where the referring physicians believed the patients to lack capacity), only 10% of the patients were threatening to leave AMA (Kornfeld 2009). Assuming psychiatrists make more accurate decision-making capacity determinations, the data suggests that nonpsychiatric physicians may be more likely to ascribe capacity to a patient with questionable capacity when that patient is attempting to leave AMA. This suggests that physicians' decision-making is influenced by powerful emotions and offers an opportunity for self-reflection about the clinical decision-making process. In such cases a psychiatric consultation may offer more than an opinion about the patient's capacity; it may offer an opportunity to reflect with a colleague as to what led and/or contributed to the AMA discharge.

Although at least briefly considering whether any patient who requests to leave the hospital AMA has the capacity to make that decision is advisable, it is important to be aware that patients with psychiatric illness or substance use disorders can still have the capacity to make medical decisions for themselves.

Conclusion

Patients requesting to leave AMA may elicit strong feelings from the treatment team. Such emotions have the potential to interfere with a clear assessment of the clinical situation and an understanding of the patient's clinical state and his/her motivations. Health-care professionals who are aware of these reactions can significantly help mitigate their impact. We recommend that physicians consider the following questions when a patient requests to leave the hospital AMA:

1. *Why is this patient signing out?*

The most important issue to consider when a patient makes an AMA request is the motivation behind the request. Some reasons are complicated and involve patient-staff dynamics, as discussed throughout this chapter, and others are more concrete and potentially more easily addressed, as discussed in other chapters.

2. *Are the patient's requests unreasonable?*

Physicians often assume that no matter could possibly be more important than the health of the patient; however, many patients do not feel the same way. When patients who are physicians behave in the same way, they may decide it is "time" for discharge over the objection of their personal physician. The patient may wish to leave to arrange childcare or pet care. This is particularly important when patients are admitted from the emergency room and were not expecting to be admitted. There may be important pending financial issues. As physicians we would like the patient to prioritize his/her medical health; sometimes these other issues are experienced as more pressing for the patient. Ideally the team can attempt to ameliorate these issues on behalf of the patient. It may be the case that the other matters cannot be resolved with the patient in the hospital and the patient's request to settle these issues before completing his or her ongoing medical treatment may not be completely unreasonable.

3. *Does the discharge need to be right now?*

Despite doing our best to understand the patient's motivation in requesting to leave AMA, when the patient requests to be discharged in the middle of the night, the physician should consider whether any other matter should actually necessitate an overnight discharge. In this case, questioning the patient's capacity to make this decision is especially relevant. The request to leave may have been on the patient's mind all day but was never discussed with the primary team. The patient might have been afraid to bring it up with his regular physician and is more comfortable speaking to someone not involved with his daily care. No matter what the underlying motivation is for the request, waiting until the "light of day" is a reasonable response to an unreasonable request to leave AMA.

4. *What are the consequences of this patient leaving AMA?*

The patient who will likely die as a consequence of leaving AMA from the hospital is very different from the patient whose team would ideally like to observe the patient for another day, but leaving 1 day early is unlikely to have any deleterious effects. A clear assessment of the consequences of an AMA discharge can help the physician decide if it is essential to attempt to block the discharge.

5. *Does this need to be an "AMA" discharge?*

Related to question 4, if the patient's hospitalization is essentially complete, barring another day of observation, the patient's discharge may not have to be "against medical advice."

6. *Do I feel relieved or angry?*

If the patient's request to leave provokes an intense emotional reaction in the treating physician, there may be some important transference/countertransference issues taking place as discussed at the beginning of this chapter. Consider whether any of these issues may be a barrier to a collaborative negotiation of the patient's concerns.

7. *Is this patient being followed by psychiatry?*

If the patient has been evaluated by psychiatry during the current admission, the psychiatric consultant may have helpful advice or input regarding the patient's request.

8. *Is there any reason to question this patient's capacity?*

If the patient seems to lack an appreciation of the need for continued admission or the consequences of an immediate discharge are severe, consider whether the patient lacks capacity to participate in discharge planning. Performing a capacity assessment is not rocket science. It is a discussion regarding the patient's understanding of the facts of the medical condition and the consequences of having or not having continued treatment. If the discussion does not provide a clear answer regarding the capacity of the patient to make informed decisions, a psychiatric consultant might be of assistance.

9. *Am I covering for the patient's primary team?*

If the patient requests to leave AMA on a weekend or overnight, it is usually advisable to consider whether a decision about discharge should be deferred to the primary team who knows the patient better. This can be accomplished by either recommending to the patient that his/her primary inpatient physician is more familiar with the case and more capable of addressing barriers to continued admission. Careful consideration of the patient's capacity should be addressed if clinically relevant.

10. *Do I need a second opinion?*

If the patient's request provokes intense emotions or the case is particularly complicated, it is never ill-advised to seek assistance from a neutral colleague or psychiatric consultant.

In general, patients with psychiatric illness are more likely to leave the hospital AMA and thus require special consideration. When in doubt about a patient's capacity to make the decision to leave AMA or when faced with a particularly difficult patient, requesting a psychiatric consult is always a useful part of the care of the patient; however, the request might be for help in managing the situation and not for "please assess capacity." There may be times when it is clear that the patient lacks capacity to make an informed decision, and leaving the hospital places the patient at risk for serious harm. Assessing the capacity of the patient should follow generally accepted principles [25]. A review of consultations requested for decision-making capacity (DMC) found that 56.8% of the consultations were "unwarranted" and the majority of such cases had neuropsychiatric disturbances [26]. In the subgroup for whom consultations were requested regarding a patient's ability to sign out AMA (21% of the total sample), more than half of the cases (18/31; 58%) were judged to be unwarranted by the investigators [26]. By unwarranted they meant, "initiated in the absence of a clearly articulated suspicion as to whether and why the patient might lack capacity." In cases where there is an obvious psychiatric disorder such as psychosis that directly impairs the ability of the patient to make a rational decision, a psychiatric consultation should be obtained. Treating a medically ill patient psychiatrically, over the patient's objection, may be required in some urgent situations to restore the patient's capacity. Hospital ethical and legal experts may be part of this decision to treat, not treat, or allow the patient to leave the hospital AMA.

References

1. Albert HD, Kornfeld DS. The threat to sign out against medical advice. Ann Intern Med. 1973;79:888–91.
2. Schlauch RW, Reich P, Kelly MJ. Leaving the hospital against advice. N Engl J Med. 1979;300:22–4.
3. Pedersen B, Oppedal K, Egund L, Tønnesen H. Will emergency and surgical patients participate in and complete alcohol interventions? A systematic review. BMC Surg. 2011;11:26.
4. Viederman M, Perry SW. Use of a psychodynamic life narrative in the treatment of depression in the physically ill. Gen Hosp Psychiatry. 1980;2(3):177–85.
5. Muskin PR. The request to die: role for a psychodynamic perspective on physician-assisted suicide. JAMA. 1998;279(4):323–8.
6. Choung AL, Joon PC, Sang CC, Hyuk HK, Ju OP. Patients who leave the emergency department against medical advice. Clin Exp Emerg Med. 2016;3(2):88–94.
7. Seaborn Moyse H, Osmun WE. Discharges against medical advice: a community hospital's experience. Can J Rural Med. 2004;9(3):148–53.
8. Saia M, Buja A, Mantoan D, Bertoncello C, Baldovin T, Callegaro G, Baldo V. Frequency and trends of hospital discharges against medical advice (DAMA) in a large administrative database. Ann Ist Super Sanita. 2014;50(4):357–62.
9. Duñó R, Pousa E, Sans J, Tolosa C, Ruiz A. Discharge against medical advice at a general hospital in Catalonia. Gen Hosp Psychiatry. 2003;25(1):46–50.
10. Holden P, Vogtsberger KN, Mohl PC, Fuller DS. Patients who leave the hospital against medical advice: the role of the psychiatric consultant. Psychosomatics. 1989;30(4):396–404.

11. Ti L, Ti L. Leaving the hospital against medical advice among people who use illicit drugs: a systematic review. Am J Public Health. 2015;105(12):e53–9.
12. Jankowski CB, Drum DE. Diagnostic correlates of discharge against medical advice. Arch Gen Psychiatry. 1977;34(2):153–5.
13. Henson VL, Vickery DS. Patient self discharge from the emergency department: who is at risk? Emerg Med J. 2005;22(7):499–501.
14. Stranges E, Weir L, Merrill CT, Steiner C. Hospitalizations in which patients leave the hospital against medical advie (AMA); 2007. Available at: http://www.hcup-us.ahrq.gov/reports/stat-briefs/sb78.pdf. May 11, 2017.
15. Alfandre DJ. "I'm going home": discharges against medical advice. Mayo Clin Proc. 2009;84(3):255–60.
16. Hwang SW, Li J, Gupta R, Chien V, Martin RE. What happens to patients who leave hospital against medical advice? CMAJ. 2003;168(4):417–20.
17. Stuppaeck CH, Barnas C, Falk M, Guenther V, Hummer M, Oberbauer H, et al. Assessment of the alcohol withdrawal syndrome – validity and reliability of the translated and modified Clinical Institute Withdrawal Assessment for Alcohol scale (CIWA-A). Addiction. 1994;89:1287–92.
18. Prochaska J, DiClemente CC, Norcross JC. In search of how people change: applications to addictive behaviors. Am Psychol. 1992;47(9):1102–14.
19. Lenounis P, Arnaout B, Marienfeld C. Motivational interviewing for clinical practice. Arlington: American Psychiatric Publishing; 2017.
20. Ness D. Discussing treatment options and risks with medical patients who have psychiatric problems. Arch Intern Med. 2002;162:2037–44.
21. Miller MC. Personality disorders. Med Clin N Am. 2001;85(3):819–37.
22. Kahana R, Bibring G. Personality types in medical management. In: Zinberg N, editor. Psychiatry and medical practice in a general hospital. New York: International Universities Press; 1964. p. 108–23.
23. Kornfeld DS, Muskin PR, Tahil FA. Psychiatric evaluation of mental capacity in the general hospital: a significant teaching opportunity. Psychosomatics. 2009;50:468–73.
24. Kahn DR, Bourgeois JA, Klein SC, Iosif AM. A prospective observational study of decisional capacity determinations in an academic medical center. Int J Psychiatry Med. 2009;39(4):405–15.
25. Appelbaum PS. Assessment of patients' competence to consent to treatment. N Engl J Med. 2007;357:1834–40.
26. Pesanti S, Hamm B, Esplin B, Karafa M, Jimenez XF. Capacity evaluation requests in the medical setting: a retrospective analysis of underlying psychosocial and ethical factors. Psychosomatics. 2017;58:483–9.

Chapter 10
Against Medical Advice Discharges: Pediatric Considerations

Armand H. Matheny Antommaria

Case

You are working the night shift and at 2:12 am you go into Jane Doe's room to admit her. Jane is an 18-day-old, term infant who is being admitted for a fever without a clear source of infection, e.g., pneumonia. She is Ms. Doe's second child, and this pregnancy and delivery were without complication. Ms. Doe tested negative for group B *streptococcus* and denies a history or symptoms of a herpes infection. She reports that Jane felt warm to the touch this morning. She took her temperature with a tympanic thermometer and it was 100.8 °F. She called Jane's pediatrician, who instructed her to bring Jane to the emergency department.

After a long wait, the physicians eventually saw Jane. They recommended a full sepsis evaluation, including blood, urine, and cerebral spinal fluid studies, and admission for empiric antibiotic therapy. Although her mother was reluctant because Jane looked well, she agreed to this plan. It took the nurse several attempts to draw blood and place an IV. The resident was unable to obtain cerebral spinal fluid after two tries, and the attending was successful on her first. Jane's white blood cell count was 10,200 per microliter with 2% bands; urinalysis was negative for nitrite and leukocyte esterase and had 2 white blood cells per high power field; and cerebral spinal fluid had 18 white blood cells and 1367 red blood cells per microliter and a negative gram stain.

On the floor, Ms. Doe looks tired. As you elicit the history, she asks why Jane needs to stay in the hospital. As you explain, Jane's nurse tries to flush her IV and reports that it has infiltrated. When she says that she will call the IV team to replace it, Ms. Doe becomes irate, states that she is tired of her daughter being used as a pin cushion, and demands to leave.

A. H. M. Antommaria (✉)
Department of Pediatrics, Cincinnati Children's Hospital Medical Center,
Cincinnati, OH, USA
e-mail: armand.antommaria@cchmc.org

© Springer International Publishing AG, part of Springer Nature 2018
D. Alfandre (ed.), *Against-Medical-Advice Discharges from the Hospital*,
https://doi.org/10.1007/978-3-319-75130-6_10

Patients may, at times, seek to be discharged against medical advice (AMA). Many institutions have policies and procedures for managing these requests, including asking patients to sign a form indicating that they understand and accept the potential risks. While educating patients about the potential risks of leaving prematurely is important, this focus may ignore the variety of reasons patients request discharge. Using the skills of principled negotiation may help health-care providers address emotional and relationship issues, identify the reasons underlying the requests, develop alternative plans that meet patients' needs, and avoid the situations from devolving into power struggles. While adult patients generally have broad discretion, there are some situations in which discharging them AMA is inappropriate. They include when patients lack medical decision-making capacity or qualify for civil commitment. In pediatrics, discharge AMA is inappropriate if doing so would constitute medical neglect. If an agreement cannot be reached and the patient should not be detained, a follow-up plan should be established. While there is no evidence that asking patients to sign an AMA form is beneficial, it may be helpful to ask patients to commit to the discharge plan.

Epidemiologic Data

Many authors characterize discharge AMA as a patient seeking to be discharged prior to their health-care providers believing that the patient is ready or it is safe [1–3]. Alfandre has emphasized the lack of standards for these discharges and proposed the following definition: "a patient request for a discharge treatment plan that is outside the range of medically acceptable options (1658) [4]." Such discharges may occur in the emergency department in addition to the inpatient setting [5–7]. Related phenomena include patients who leave prior to being seen by a medical provider [6] and patients who leave without notifying their health-care providers [8]. Empirical studies of these phenomena vary in their inclusion and exclusion criteria.

Patients seeking to be discharged AMA is a relatively common occurrence. The frequency varies by health-care setting and diagnosis. The rate for hospitalized, general medical patients in the United States and Canada is 1–2% [9–11]. The rate is higher for psychiatric patients (3–51%) [12], patients who abuse drugs or alcohol (5.3%) [13], and patients with human immunodeficiency virus (HIV) infections (13%) [14]. The rate may be increasing over time. Stranges et al. report a 39% increase in discharges AMA between 1997 and 2007 [10, 11].

Researchers have attempted to identify sociodemographic factors associated with discharge AMA. The quality of this literature varies. Studies have examined different lists of factors and some studies only report univariate analyses [8]. The strongest predictor of discharge AMA is prior discharge AMA [10, 15]. Other potential factors include younger age, male gender, lower income, and public or no health insurance [11, 16, 17]. The data regarding whether discharge AMA is associated with race is inconsistent [9, 16, 17].

The results of these studies, however, do not permit sufficiently accurate prediction of patients likely to seek discharge AMA to target interventions. There are few intervention studies, and most have been conducted in psychiatric facilities where the rate of discharges AMA is higher. Targum et al., for example, describes the implementation of a patient advocate who oriented new patients, addressed misconceptions, and acted as an intermediary with the staff. They report a reduction in AMA discharges from 11.2% to 7.6% ($p < 0.01$) [18].

Discharge AMA is typically defined relative to the health-care providers' perceptions or predictions. The available data suggests that these predictions have some validity; patients discharged AMA have higher readmission and mortality rates. Southern et al., for example, conducted a retrospective cohort study of general medical inpatients at Montefiore Medical Center, Bronx, New York, from July 1, 2002 to June 30, 2008. There were 3544 (2.4% of total admissions) discharges AMA and 80,536 (54.1%) planned discharges during this time. To control for confounding, the authors used logistic regression modeling and propensity score matching. In the matched analysis, patients discharged AMA had a higher 30-day readmission rate (OR 1.65, 95% CI 1.46–1.87) and 30-day mortality rate (OR 2.46, 95% CI 1.29–4.68) [19]. These results are consistent with those of other studies of general medical patients [3, 8, 9] and specific patient populations [16, 20, 21].

One study also examined the length of stay upon readmission. Anis et al. studied patients with HIV admitted to St. Paul's Hospital, Vancouver. In multivariate analysis, they found that length of stay upon readmission was longer for patients discharged AMA compared to patients discharged formally. The log scale of the ratio of the length of stay of patients discharged AMA to patients discharged formally was 0.34 (95% CI 0.04–0.63) [14]. This study suggests that patients who are discharged AMA have unresolved health-care needs at discharge that may worsen while an outpatient.

There is very limited data available about pediatric discharges AMA in the United States or Canada. Reinke et al. conducted a retrospective medical record review of patients presenting to St. Louis Children's Hospital Emergency Department from January 1, 1999 to December 31, 2003. During this time, 250 (0.1%) patients were discharged AMA including 20 patients who left without being seen and 93 who eloped. They found age 15–20 years (OR 4.200, 95% CI 1.100–16.200) and arrival by ambulance (OR 2.428, 95% CI 9.950–10.001) were positively associated with discharge AMA, and triage category urgent (OR 0.039, 95% CI 0.002–0.653) and several discharge diagnoses were negatively associated. In unadjusted analyses, a higher percentage of patients discharged AMA returned to the emergency department within 15 days (24.5% vs. 6.4%, $p < 0.001$). A higher percentage of patients who were discharged AMA also returned for the same complaint (95.7% vs 50.0%, $p = 0.003$), but a similar percentage were admitted to the hospital (25%) [7]. I was, however, unable to identify any other pediatric studies in the United States or Canada, and it is difficult to generalize from a single study.

Pediatric studies have been conducted in other countries including India [22], Iran [23], and Nigeria [24]. It is not clear what accounts for this difference in interest in this topic. For example, the rate of discharge AMA from the neonatal intensive care unit at the Shree Krishna Hospital, Gujarat, India, was 25.4% [22].

Policies and Procedures

Institutions generally have procedures for discharging patients AMA. They entail disclosing the risks of discharge and documenting the understanding of these risks. Patients may be asked to sign a specific form (Fig. 10.1). Unfortunately, there are no studies of the frequency or content of these policies. The exception is Schaefer et al.'s description of the frequency with which a convenience sample of forms includes mention of potential financial consequences of leaving AMA [25].

The conventional approach has some potential benefits. Patients' decisions should be informed. While efforts to educate patients should occur throughout their hospitalizations, patients may not sufficiently understand their diagnoses, treatments, and potential risks of leaving at the time they request discharge. Describing the potential risks may increase the likelihood that patients' decisions are adequately informed.

Some providers believe that one of the potential risks of discharge AMA is that insurers will not pay for the hospitalization and that patients may become responsible for the entire bill. Schaefer et al. performed an analysis of a subgroup of general medical patients who were enrolled in a larger study at the University of Chicago Hospital between July 2001 and March 2010. One percent of patients (526/46,319) were discharged AMA. Insurance companies denied payment 4.0% of the time, and there was no instance in which an insurance company denied payment because the patient had been discharged AMA. (Few patients (9.7%), however, had private insurance which limits the generalizability of these results [25].) Conveying that patients might bear financial responsibility if they leave AMA may, therefore, be inaccurate. Such claims should not be used to coerce patients into staying [1, 4].

The rationale for asking patients to sign a form is not clear. One might argue that asking patients to do this reinforces the significance of the decision. There is, however, no direct evidence that asking patients to sign a form improves their understanding or decreases the rate of discharge AMA [26].

The psychology literature suggests that individuals strongly associate their signatures with their identities and that signing your name acts as a general self-identity prime. Signing your name activates the aspect of your self-identity relevant to the situation and produces behavior congruent with this aspect of your self-identity. Kettle and Haubl, for example, showed that individuals who self-identified as runners were more engaged in shopping for a pair of running shoes after signing their names [27]. It is not, however, clear in the context of discharge AMA what aspects of self-identity are activated. Having patients sign their names might decrease or increase the number of discharges depending on which aspect is primed.

Name:_____

MRN:_____ DOB:_____

Patient _____ Date_____ Time_____

I, _____ demand that XXXXX Children's Hospital release me/my child _____ (relationship), against the advice and recommendation of the physician and I therefore assume full responsibility for any harm that may arise from this action.

Dr. _____ has fully discussed and completely explained the seriousness of my/my child's medical problem. I am fully aware that I/my child has been diagnosed with

_____

_____

____

and that

_____

_____

____

are the reasonably expected complications that could arise as a result of my choice to discontinue treatment here at the medical center. Details of the surgical, medical or diagnostic services that could be rendered to me/my child here within the medical center, their purpose and possible results have been explained fully to my satisfaction.

I understand that the medical center releases me/my child reluctantly and against the medical advice and recommendations of its medical staff.

I ACKNOWLEDGE THAT ALL OF THE INFORMATION GIVEN TO ME RECOMMENDS AND ADVISES THAT I NOT REMOVE MYSELF/MY CHILD FROM THE MEDICAL CENTER. I understand the nature, seriousness and extent of the medical problem of me/my child and even in light of all the information I have received and the information that is contained within this form, I hereby order the medical center to release me/my child against medical advice.

Witness _____ Time/Date _____

Witness _____ Time/Date _____

Signature _____ Relationship _____

Fig. 10.1 Example of a release against medical advice form

Some providers may also believe that having patients sign discharge AMA forms creates legal immunities. Signed forms are, however, neither sufficient nor necessary documentation of the interaction. Forms that release providers from all future liability have generally not been upheld by the courts. A signature on a discharge form

Table 10.1 Required components of a comprehensive against medical advice form and discharge instructions

Formalities
Signature of physician and patient
Date and time of against medical advice discussion and form execution
Personalized to patient
Medical condition(s)
Specific risks and benefits of proposed treatment and alternatives
Specific consequences of leaving against medical advice
Reports results of mental capacity assessment
Patient understanding of proposed treatment
Patient understanding of consequences of refusing treatment
Patient's reason for refusal of admission or treatment
Lists follow-up instructions
Self-care and when to seek medical attention
Arrangements with police, social services, relatives, etc.

Reprinted from Levy et al. [28], with permission from Elsevier

also does not, in and of itself, guarantee adequately informed consent [28]. For example, in *Battenfeld v. Gregory*, the jury found against two emergency medicine physicians, although the patient had signed a discharge AMA form, because they did not inform the patient of the risks [29]. Poorly written forms may give providers false reassurance that they have fulfilled the requirements [1].

There are also potential limitations and risks of asking patients to sign discharge AMA forms. Forms may not be written at an appropriate reading level [4]. The sample form reproduced in Fig. 10.1, for example, is written at greater than the twelfth grade reading level. Some of its language, e.g., "I demand" and "I hereby order," also characterizes the patient or parent's actions in negative ways. The language "fully" and "all" may overstate the situation. Asking individuals to sign discharge AMA forms may unintentionally exacerbate the conflict.

The encounter should be documented in the patient's medical record. This can, however, be done without the use of a specialized form. There is nonetheless evidence that providers inadequately document these encounters [5]. Use of a comprehensive AMA form [30], or template or dot phrase, may increase the likelihood that all relevant information is included (Table 10.1). While appropriately documenting the encounter may not prevent a lawsuit, it can provide several potential defenses should one arise, e.g., the duty to treat had ended [28].

Principled Negotiation

Although informing patients of the benefits of continued hospitalization and the risks of discharge, and documenting the encounters, has potential benefits, this approach is nonetheless limited. Patients seek to be discharged for a variety of reasons including feeling better, family concerns or obligations, work or financial obligations, and dissatisfaction with care [8, 15, 16, 18]. (The international studies of pediatric populations identify additional reasons. Jimoh et al., for example, report 32.6% of parents cited financial constraints directly related to the cost of treatment and 17.7% the desire to seek alternative therapy including traditional bonesetters or birth attendants [24].) Discussing the risks may address the concerns of patients who feel better, but does not address these other issues.

I would argue that patients' request for discharge should be interpreted as initiating a negotiation and that providers should be trained in and utilize negotiation skills to address these requests. This is consistent with Clark et al.'s practical approach [1], Alfandre's emphasis on patient-centered care and shared decision-making [4, 26], and Saitz's emphasis on physician-patient communication [31]. Negotiation is a form of conflict resolution that involves the parties themselves. Alternatives include resorting to violence or involving a third party. The forms of third party conflict resolution differ in terms of the third party's authority. In mediation, the third party facilitates the interaction between the principal parties but does not have authority to impose a settlement. In contrast, in litigation, a judge has authority to impose a binding outcome [32]. The use of a third party in discharges AMA may not be feasible given the urgency of the requests. If it is, family relations staff, social workers, and/or clinical ethics consultants may be able to help.

One approach to negotiation is principled negotiation, which can be contrasted with positional bargaining. In positional bargaining, the parties assert positions, argue for them, make concessions, and potentially reach a compromise. Positions are concrete, tangible outcomes of the negotiation [33]. In negotiations regarding discharge, positions might be the duration of hospitalization. For example, in the febrile infant case, the standard of care is to provide empiric antibiotic treatment until the blood, urine, and cerebrospinal fluid cultures have incubated for 36 h [34]. The parent might demand immediate discharge and the provider assert that the patient needs to remain hospitalized for 36 h.

A limitation of positional bargaining is that participants tend to identify themselves with, and lock themselves into, their positions. Agreement may become less likely, and if it occurs, it may be the result of splitting the difference between positions [33]. In our example, the provider might compromise and state that he/she would be willing to discharge Jane after 24 h. Arguing over positions may also become a battle of wills and damage the relationship between the parties [33]. If the encounter becomes acrimonious, Ms. Doe may be less likely to inquire about medical concerns in the future. If one party makes concessions to maintain the relationship, it increases the likelihood of an unwise outcome [33].

Table 10.2 Principled
negotiation

Participants are problem-solvers
The goal is a wise outcome reached efficiently and amicably
Separate the people from the problems
Be soft on the people, hard on the problem
Proceed independent of trust
Focus on interests, not positions
Explore interests
Avoid having a bottom line
Invent options for mutual gain
Develop multiple options to choose from; decide later
Insist on using objective criteria
Try to reach a result based on standards independent of will
Reason and be open to reason; yield to principle, not pressure

In contrast, principled negotiation has four components: separating the people from the problem, focusing on interests, expanding the options before evaluating them, and appealing to objective standards [33] (Table 10.2).

Separating the people from the problem means addressing the emotional and relationship issues separately from the substantive issues [33]. Even if the provider is a hospitalist and does not have an ongoing personal relationship with the patient, it is important to maintain a positive relationship with the patient and family. The provider does not want the parents to forego well-child care or delay seeking treatment for acute issues due to a prior negative experience.

There are a variety of ways to address the emotional and relationship issues. One way is to avoid blaming the other party for your problem. Even if justified, it is likely to make the other party defensive and may encourage them to counterattack [33]. In this situation, the admitting provider may be tired or may have other patients to see. Suggesting that Ms. Doe is taking up an inordinate amount of his/her time is likely to be counterproductive. In addition to recognizing and understanding emotions, it is valuable to make them explicit and acknowledge them as legitimate [33]. Ms. Doe may be experiencing a variety of emotions including fatigue, frustration, and anger. The provider might state, "You look tired. I am sorry that you have had such a long day and it is so late." Patients may need to be able to express their frustration, and it is important to not react to emotional outbursts. This may entail actively listening to their grievances including restating or paraphrasing them [33]. The provider might summarize, "I want to be sure that I understand you correctly: Jane is acting normally and you are concerned that starting a new IV will be painful and unnecessary." Restating or paraphrasing the concern provides the opportunity to correct misunderstandings. One of the goals is for the parties to reorient, to see themselves as working side-by-side to solve a shared problem [33].

Interests are the needs, desires, concerns, and fears that underlie positions. They include security, financial stability, a sense of community, and control [33]. In the health-care context, a position might be the discharge date and time, while the underlying interest might be the patient returning to school or the parent maintaining his/her job. In our case, Ms. Doe may have a variety of interests: assuring Jane's health, protecting Jane from unnecessary pain, and obtaining rest for Jane and herself. She might also have an interest assuring that her older son gets off to preschool safely and/or keeping her job. One way to help identify interests is to consider or ask why the other party favors or disfavors a position. Focusing on interests is important because an interest may be satisfied by several positions, and the parties may have shared and differing but complementary interests, in addition to conflicting ones [33]. Patients, parents, and providers, for example, generally share an interest in promoting patients' health. The admitting provider's interest in admitting his/her next patient and Ms. Doe's interest in going to sleep are potentially compatible.

Often individuals approach negotiations as though the outcome is a fixed pie— for someone to get more, someone else must receive less. This is not always the case. It may be possible to expand the pie, to invent options that are advantageous to both/all parties, before dividing it [33]. Alfandre acknowledges that a medically safe treatment plan "potentially includes more than just the single treatment option of remaining hospitalized (1660) [4]." In the febrile infant case, other options might include monitoring the patient in the hospital without administering antibiotics, or administering the antibiotics intramuscularly. Techniques for expanding options include brainstorming and the circle chart. Unfortunately, premature judgment or criticism, and searching for the single answer, may inhibit generating a variety of options [33].

Finally, when evaluating the options, it is beneficial to appeal to fair or objective standards rather than base the choice on will, pressure, or threats [33]. For example, a health-care provider might appeal to a professional society's care practice guideline or offer a second, independent opinion. In Jane Doe's case, objective standards might include evidence of risks of withholding antibiotics, or the incremental benefits of longer empiric antibiotic therapy. In this case, the risk of a serious bacterial infection is approximately 15% [35], and the rate that cultures turn positive decreases with time [36]. Objective standards can also be used to select among multiple standards. In other contexts, one might have to rely on a fair procedure such as letting someone else decide. Using objective standards allows individuals who change their positions to appear reasonable rather than weak. Individuals may become invested in their positions, and it may be important to give them the opportunity to back down gracefully. Requiring sound reasons generally has greater legitimacy and persuasiveness, and refusing to yield to pressure is usually a stronger position to defend [33].

In the Jane Doe example, the admitting provider might convey that the members of the IV team are very experienced in placing IVs in children. He/she might try to negotiate allowing them to try one or two times. If this is not successful, he/she might try to convince Ms. Doe to remain in the hospital for 24 h for observation. This position would be another way to meet the shared interest in promoting Jane's health. Depending on Ms. Doe's dominant interests, he/she might also seek to put off a final decision until after Ms. Doe has had a chance to sleep, or to convince her that it is alright to leave her daughter in the hospital while she goes home to get her son ready for school. She could call in at any time to check on Jane, and the nursing staff will call her if there are significant changes in Jane's condition. These positions would attempt to address Ms. Doe's independent interests.

Medical Neglect

In negotiation, not reaching an agreement is always a possibility and might be the best option. Agreements should be evaluated against the best alternative to a negotiated agreement (BATNA). Comparing the offer to the BATNA can protect participants from accepting unfavorable offers or rejecting favorable ones [33].

Adult patients generally have wide discretion in medical decision-making. Adults with medical decision-making capacity, for example, may refuse life-sustaining medical treatment. There are, nonetheless, some limitations on patients' ability to leave AMA. These include lacking medical decision-making capacity [28] or fulfilling the requirements for civil commitment [37]. Having capacity requires the ability to understand the potential benefits, risks, and alternatives of the proposed treatment, the ability to appreciate the implications for one's own life, the ability to evaluate the potential benefits and risks, and the ability to express a preference. Capacity is relative to the decision being made, and the threshold may be higher for more complex decisions. In many situations, internists are competent to determine whether patients possess capacity. There is, unfortunately, no simple, accurate test for capacity. In more difficult cases, consultation with a specialist, e.g., a psychiatrist, may be beneficial [28].

Conversely, adolescents should be incorporated in medical decision-making based on the level of their developing capacity. The different components of capacity typically develop at different ages. While 16- or 17-year-olds may have the capacity to understand, they may not be sufficiently able to appreciate or evaluate the information. Even if they possess adequate medical decision-making capacity, minors do not generally have the legal authority to provide informed consent including discharging themselves AMA. Disagreement between children and their parents may make situations even more complex. Providers may require others' assistance, e.g., clinical ethics consultants, social workers, and/or risk managers, to adequately address such situations [38].

In adult medicine, another reason to refuse to discharge patients AMA is that they fulfill the criteria for civil commitment [37]. All states permit health-care providers to temporarily detain patients who are at a significant, immediate risk of harming themselves or others. There is debate over whether other criteria, such as inability to care for oneself, are also appropriate [39].

In pediatrics, parents generally have wide discretion in making decisions for their children. This serves several important societal goals. Families are the primary social institutions for rearing children [40]. Parents are often best situated to understand their children's interests and make decisions for them. They also bear the consequences of the decisions. Finally, limiting oversight and intrusion provides families the space and freedom they require to flourish [41].

This discretion is not, however, unlimited [40, 41]. Under the doctrine of *parens patriae*, the state is justified in intervening to protect the life and health of those who cannot care for themselves [42, 43]. The state may also use its police powers to punish individuals guilty of child abuse or neglect, e.g., parents whose children die as the result of a lack of medically indicated treatment can be charged with felony child abuse, negligent homicide, and/or manslaughter [44].

There is ongoing debate within pediatric bioethics about how best to conceptualize the threshold for state intervention in parental decision-making [45]. The general standard for parental decision-making is the best interest standard—"acting so as to promote maximally the good of the individual (88) [46]." There are general criticisms of this standard including difficulties determining what is in a child's best interests and the legitimacy of other family members' and the family as a whole's interests. Simply acting inconsistent with a child's best interests is generally not considered a sufficient justification for intervention. It is difficult to determine how large a deviation is necessary. Kopelman, for example, argues that the best interest standard is only relevant to determining how to intervene [47].

The most common standard focuses on harm to the child. Diekema argues that state intervention is justified if the refusal places the child at significant and imminent risk of serious harm, the proposed intervention is likely to prevent this harm, and the benefits of the proposed intervention outweighs the harm of restricting parental choice. He enumerates several additional criteria including that state intervention is necessary and the least restrictive alternative [43] (Table 10.3). Some other authors focus on the rationality of the decision instead [48].

The paradigmatic case of medical neglect is parents who are Jehovah's Witnesses and who refuse a potentially lifesaving blood transfusion for their child. The patient's anemia may be so severe as to pose a significant and imminent risk of death, and a transfusion may be lifesaving if the anemia can be treated. In emergencies, providers should treat and, in situations in which time permits, they should seek a court order prior to treating. Cases such as chemotherapy or solid organ transplantation may be less clear. The risk of nontreatment may not be imminent, and the treatment may have limited efficacy and serious side effects. Because these are ongoing treatments, the interventions required to effectuate them, e.g., placing the child in a medical foster home, may cause substantial harm. State intervention may, therefore, not be justified [43].

Table 10.3 Conditions for justified state interference with parental decision-making

1. By refusing to consent are the parents placing their child at significant risk of serious harm?
2. Is the harm imminent, requiring immediate action to prevent it?
3. Is the intervention that has been refused necessary to prevent the serious harm?
4. Is the intervention that has been refused of proven efficacy and, therefore, likely to prevent the harm?
5. Does the intervention that has been refused by the parents not also place the child at significant risk of serious harm, and do its projected benefits outweigh its projected burdens significantly more favorably than the option chosen by the parents?
6. Would any other option prevent serious harm to the child in a way that is less intrusive to parental autonomy and more acceptable to the parents?
7. Can the state intervention be generalized to all other similar situations?
8. Would most parents agree that the state intervention was reasonable?

Diekema [43]

In the febrile infant case, taking the patient home without further antibiotic therapy is unlikely to constitute medical neglect. The risk of a serious bacterial infection is approximately 15%, and, even if the patient has a serious bacterial infection and becomes sicker, there is likely to be an opportunity to intervene to prevent permanent harm. The admitting provider's BATNA, i.e., discharge, is relatively poor, and the provider has a significant incentive to negotiate. In contrast, if Jane was persistently febrile, was ill appearing with a bulging fontanelle, and had an elevated cerebral spinal fluid white blood cell count and protein, a low glucose, and a positive gram stain, the likelihood of bacterial meningitis, and therefore the chance of dying or becoming seriously disabled if untreated, would be substantially higher. Even continued hospitalization without antibiotic therapy would likely constitute medical neglect. The provider's BATNA, i.e., a court order mandating treatment, is relatively high, and he/she would be justified in not making concessions regarding discharge. He/she might, nonetheless, seek to address the emotional and relationship issues, and Ms. Doe's other interests.

Discharge

If a negotiated agreement cannot be reached, and an adult patient possesses capacity and does not fulfill the criteria for civil commitment or a pediatric patient's discharge does not constitute medical neglect, providers are obligated to discharge patients. They should pay significant attention to post-discharge management [1, 2, 4, 21, 49]. This planning may be difficult because patients discharged AMA are more likely not to have a primary care provider [17]. Discharge planning includes providing the most effective treatment, describing the reasons parents should seek medical attention, and scheduling follow-up care. Withholding beneficial but less effective treatment may constitute coercion [50]. In Jane's case, the provider might recommend a dose of intramuscular antibiotics. He/she might encourage Ms. Doe to follow up with Jane's primary care provider within 24 h, and call the primary care provider so that he/she will contact Ms. Doe if she does not follow up.

It is at this point that requesting patients sign a document, e.g., a discharge plan, might be beneficial. Signing a document influences behavior pertinent to the document. For example, postmenopausal African American women who signed a behavioral contract were more likely to adhere to a brisk walking goal [51]. While a discharge plan does not have all the components of a behavioral contract, e.g., it lacks rewards [32], it might nonetheless be beneficial to request patients sign a document committing them to appropriate follow up.

Conclusions

Discharges AMA have historically focused on informing patients of the risks of discharge and documenting their acceptance of these risks. This narrow scope ignores the diversity of reasons that patients seek to be discharged AMA. It is potentially beneficial to use principled negotiation to identify patients' interests and negotiate a mutually acceptable treatment plan. If this fails, providers should assure that discharge does not constitute medical neglect and promote appropriate follow-up care.

References

1. Clark MA, Abbott JT, Adyanthaya T. Ethics seminars: a best-practice approach to navigating the against-medical-advice discharge. Acad Emerg Med. 2014;21(9):1050–7.
2. Defillippis EM. When patients leave 'against medical advice.' The New York Times. Jan 12, 2017.
3. Yong TY, Fok JS, Hakendorf P, Ben-Tovim D, Thompson CH, Li JY. Characteristics and outcomes of discharges against medical advice among hospitalised patients. Intern Med J. 2013;43(7):798–802.
4. Alfandre D. Reconsidering against medical advice discharges: embracing patient-centeredness to promote high quality care and a renewed research agenda. J Gen Intern Med. 2013;28(12):1657–62.
5. Dubow D, Propp D, Narasimhan K. Emergency department discharges against medical advice. J Emerg Med. 1992;10(4):513–6.
6. Jerrard DA, Chasm RM. Patients leaving against medical advice (AMA) from the emergency department – disease prevalence and willingness to return. J Emerg Med. 2011;41(4):412–7.
7. Reinke DA, Walker M, Boslaugh S, Hodge D 3rd. Predictors of pediatric emergency patients discharged against medical advice. Clin Pediatr (Phila). 2009;48(3):263–70.
8. Hwang SW, Li J, Gupta R, Chien V, Martin RE. What happens to patients who leave hospital against medical advice? CMAJ. 2003;168(4):417–20.
9. Glasgow JM, Vaughn-Sarrazin M, Kaboli PJ. Leaving against medical advice (AMA): risk of 30-day mortality and hospital readmission. J Gen Intern Med. 2010;25(9):926–9.

10. Kraut A, Fransoo R, Olafson K, Ramsey CD, Yogendran M, Garland A. A population-based analysis of leaving the hospital against medical advice: incidence and associated variables. BMC Health Serv Res. 2013;13:415.
11. Stranges E, Wier L, Merrill CT, Steiner C. Hospitalizations in which patients leave the hospital against medical advice (AMA), 2007: statistical brief #78. Healthcare Cost and Utilization Project (HCUP) Statistical Briefs. Rockville, MD; 2006.
12. Brook M, Hilty DM, Liu W, Hu R, Frye MA. Discharge against medical advice from inpatient psychiatric treatment: a literature review. Psychiatr Serv. 2006;57(8):1192–8.
13. Green P, Watts D, Poole S, Dhopesh V. Why patients sign out against medical advice (AMA): factors motivating patients to sign out AMA. Am J Drug Alcohol Abuse. 2004;30(2):489–93.
14. Anis AH, Sun H, Guh DP, Palepu A, Schechter MT, O'Shaughnessy MV. Leaving hospital against medical advice among HIV-positive patients. CMAJ. 2002;167(6):633–7.
15. Jeremiah J, O'Sullivan P, Stein MD. Who leaves against medical advice? J Gen Intern Med. 1995;10(7):403–5.
16. Baptist AP, Warrier I, Arora R, Ager J, Massanari RM. Hospitalized patients with asthma who leave against medical advice: characteristics, reasons, and outcomes. J Allergy Clin Immunol. 2007;119(4):924–9.
17. Weingart SN, Davis RB, Phillips RS. Patients discharged against medical advice from a general medicine service. J Gen Intern Med. 1998;13(8):568–71.
18. Targum SD, Capodanno AE, Hoffman HA, Foudraine C. An intervention to reduce the rate of hospital discharges against medical advice. Am J Psychiatry. 1982;139(5):657–9.
19. Southern WN, Nahvi S, Arnsten JH. Increased risk of mortality and readmission among patients discharged against medical advice. Am J Med. 2012;125(6):594–602.
20. Choi M, Kim H, Qian H, Palepu A. Readmission rates of patients discharged against medical advice: a matched cohort study. PLoS One. 2011;6(9):e24459.
21. Fiscella K, Meldrum S, Barnett S. Hospital discharge against advice after myocardial infarction: deaths and readmissions. Am J Med. 2007;120(12):1047–53.
22. Devpura B, Bhadesia P, Nimbalkar S, Desai S, Phatak A. Discharge against medical advice at neonatal intensive care unit in Gujarat. India Int J Pediatr. 2016;2016:1897039.
23. Mohseni M, Alikhani M, Tourani S, Azami-Aghdash S, Royani S, Moradi-Joo M. Rate and causes of discharge against medical advice in Iranian hospitals: a systematic review and meta-analysis. Iran J Public Health. 2015;44(7):902–12.
24. Jimoh BM, Anthonia OC, Chinwe I, Oluwafemi A, Ganiyu A, Haroun A, et al. Prospective evaluation of cases of discharge against medical advice in Abuja. Nigeria Sci World J. 2015;2015:314817.
25. Schaefer GR, Matus H, Schumann JH, Sauter K, Vekhter B, Meltzer DO, et al. Financial responsibility of hospitalized patients who left against medical advice: medical urban legend? J Gen Intern Med. 2012;27(7):825–30.
26. Alfandre D, Schumann JH. What is wrong with discharges against medical advice (and how to fix them). JAMA. 2013;310(22):2393–4.
27. Kettle KL, Haubl G. The signature effect: signing influences consumption-related behavior by priming self-identity. J Constr Res. 2011;38:474–89.
28. Levy F, Mareiniss DP, Iacovelli C. The importance of a proper against-medical-advice (AMA) discharge: how signing out AMA may create significant liability protection for providers. J Emerg Med. 2012;43(3):516–20.
29. Battenfeld v. Gregory, 589 A2d 1059 (N.J. Super. Ct. App. Div. 1991).
30. Henson VL, Vickery DS. Patient self discharge from the emergency department: who is at risk? Emerg Med J. 2005;22(7):499–501.
31. Saitz R. Discharges against medical advice: time to address the causes. CMAJ. 2002;167(6):647–8.
32. Janz NK, Becker MH, Hartman PE. Contingency contracting to enhance patient compliance: a review. Patient Educ Couns. 1984;5(4):165–78.

33. Fisher R, Ury W, Bruce P. Getting to YES: negotiating agreement without giving in. 2nd ed. New York: Houghton Mifflin; 1991.
34. Arora R, Mahajan P. Evaluation of child with fever without source: review of literature and update. Pediatr Clin N Am. 2013;60(5):1049–62.
35. Watt K, Waddle E, Jhaveri R. Changing epidemiology of serious bacterial infections in febrile infants without localizing signs. PLoS One. 2010;5(8):e12448.
36. Biondi EA, Mischler M, Jerardi KE, Statile AM, French J, Evans R, et al. Blood culture time to positivity in febrile infants with bacteremia. JAMA Pediatr. 2014;168(9):844–9.
37. Devitt PJ, Devitt AC, Dewan M. An examination of whether discharging patients against medical advice protects physicians from malpractice charges. Psychiatr Serv. 2000;51(7):899–902.
38. Katz AL, Webb SA, Committee On Bioethics. Informed consent in decision-making in pediatric practice. Pediatrics. 2016;138(2):e20161485.
39. Testa M, West SG. Civil commitment in the United States. Psychiatry (Edgmont). 2010;7(10):30–40.
40. Jenny C. Committee on child abuse and neglect. Recognizing and responding to medical neglect. Pediatrics. 2007;120(6):1385–9.
41. Committee on Bioethics. Conflicts between religious or spiritual beliefs and pediatric care: informed refusal, exemptions, and public funding. Pediatrics. 2013;132(5):962–5.
42. Areen J. Intervention between parent and child: a reappraisal of the state's role in child neglect and abuse cases. Geo L J. 1975;63:887–937.
43. Diekema DS. Parental refusals of medical treatment: the harm principle as threshold for state intervention. Theor Med Bioeth. 2004;25(4):243–64.
44. Hickey KS, Lyckholm L. Child welfare versus parental autonomy: medical ethics, the law, and faith-based healing. Theor Med Bioeth. 2004;25(4):265–76.
45. McDougall RJ, Notini L. Overriding parents' medical decisions for their children: a systematic review of normative literature. J Med Ethics. 2014;40(7):448–52.
46. Buchanan AE, Brock DW. Deciding for others: the ethics of surrogate decision making. Cambridge: Cambridge University Press; 1990.
47. Kopelman LM. The best-interests standard as threshold, ideal, and standard of reasonableness. J Med Philos. 1997;22(3):271–89.
48. Rhodes R, Holzman IR. The not unreasonable standard for assessment of surrogates and surrogate decisions. Theor Med Bioeth. 2004;25(4):367–85.
49. Swota AH. Changing policy to reflect a concern for patients who sign out against medical advice. Am J Bioeth. 2007;7(3):32–4.
50. Berger JT. Discharge against medical advice: ethical considerations and professional obligations. J Hosp Med. 2008;3(5):403–8.
51. Williams BR, Bezner J, Chesbro SB, Leavitt R. The effect of a walking program on perceived benefits and barriers to exercise in postmenopausal African American women. J Geriatr Phys Ther. 2006;29(2):43–9.

Chapter 11
Against Medical Advice Discharges: Considerations in the Psychiatric Population

Cynthia Geppert

Introduction and Background

Upon first thought, discharge AMA seems to be an oxymoron when applied to inpatient psychiatric units. After all, the treatment these patients are receiving is primarily *psychiatric* and not *medical,* and frequently these are patients admitted to locked facilities involuntarily, so how can they be discharged at their request or even demand? This chapter will examine these apparent contradictions and show that the concept of AMA discharge from an inpatient psychiatry ward has substantive clinical and legal differences that in turn generate unique ethical dilemmas when compared to discharges from medical facilities. In fact, it is not clear if the AMA discharge in psychiatric settings is an administrative event or entity that meets precise criteria for AMA discharge as is understood in other sectors of hospital care.

Yet, there are obviously patients whom the literature reports as being discharged AMA from psychiatric facilities. Most of these reports are primarily demographic studies that do not either specifically define the term or describe the exact legal circumstances of the patients classified as leaving AMA. Using a strict definition as described elsewhere in this book, when a voluntary patient in a psychiatric facility on a staff walk simply runs away, this would not be counted as an AMA discharge. Such a departure is better classified as an elopement or irregular discharge or some other term depending on the facility [1]. But utilizing a looser interpretation of the term, some articles lump together elopements, administrative discharges for rule infractions, and AMA discharges [2].

C. Geppert (✉)
University of New Mexico School of Medicine, Albuquerque, NM, USA

Alden March Bioethics Institute, Albany Medical College, Albany, NY, USA
e-mail: ethicdoc@comcast.net

© Springer International Publishing AG, part of Springer Nature 2018
D. Alfandre (ed.), *Against-Medical-Advice Discharges from the Hospital,*
https://doi.org/10.1007/978-3-319-75130-6_11

One reason for this lack of specificity in definition may be because many of the articles published about AMA discharge from inpatient psychiatry were written in the 1960s and 1970s before the full community impact of the massive deinstitutionalization of psychiatric patients was appreciated [3] or in the 1980s prior to the broad penetration of managed care into mental health. These two social and economic phenomena along with the cultural change in the policy approaches to the mentally ill shape the understanding of AMA discharge examined in this chapter. Steady trends [3] in psychiatric treatment toward stricter commitment laws resulting in more voluntary admissions [4] and shorter length of stays for sicker patients have led to a "revolving door" syndrome [5] of which AMA discharges are an often neglected aspect of mental health policy and practice [6].

Epidemiology of AMA Discharges from Inpatient Psychiatry

Like the body of research on AMA discharges from general hospitals [7], studies of discharges AMA from psychiatric units have focused almost exclusively on predictive and descriptive factors [8, 9]. Of patients who choose to leave an inpatient unit before their practitioners believes it is clinically appropriate, there is relatively less attention given to either the reasons patients leave or interventions that could prevent premature departures or improve the clinical management.

Brook et al., in 2006, published the most comprehensive review of the literature on AMA discharges from inpatient psychiatry units available at the time this chapter was written [10]. The review analyzed the prevalence, predictors, temporal patterns, consequences, and interventions related to AMA discharges over the last 50 years. Searching the two largest databases of psychiatric literature, PubMed and PsychINFO, the authors identified 61 articles that met their search criteria of an article focusing on AMA discharge from an inpatient psychiatric unit as either an aim or result of the article, and that included a formal statistical analysis. Prevalence of AMA discharges ranged from 3% to 51% with the percentage increasing in articles published later compared to those written earlier.

Table 11.1 summarizes the predictive factors for AMA discharge from inpatient psychiatry units identified in multiple studies, many of which mirror those characterizing patients discharged AMA from general medical wards [11].

Several of these *patient-related* factors are not promising targets for positive interventions and would be traits associated with challenging patients in the minds of most experienced clinicians. But unlike prior studies, this review goes farther and examines *provider-related* factors that transform these encounters into difficult *provider-patient* interactions or relationships. The dyadic considerations present more promising opportunities for performance improvement in the management of patients likely to leave AMA from psychiatric units. Patients are more likely to leave AMA if they are dissatisfied with the hospitalization, view psychiatry in general, or their own treatment punitively or pessimistically which may reflect earlier negative experiences with mental health care.

Table 11.1 Patient predictive factors for AMA discharge from inpatient psychiatry

Younger (age 20s and 30s) [12, 13]
Single
Male gender
Comorbid personality disorder
Comorbid substance use disorder
Pessimistic attitude toward treatment
Antisocial personality disorder
Aggressive or disruptive behavior
History of multiple prior AMA discharges from psychiatry units

Patients were more likely to leave when they did not receive a proper and timely orientation to the psychiatric hospitalization or when the treatment team was unable or unwilling to establish a therapeutic treatment relationship or outside daytime duty hours such as on evening or weekend shifts. Several studies identified distinct cohorts such as patients who leave early and late in a hospital course or those who leave AMA only once or repeatedly that need additional replication and explication [14, 15].

Outcome and Impact on Health-Care Quality

The Brook review identified 14 articles that examined a variety of outcome parameters of AMA [10]. The readmission and mortality rates of patients leaving AMA from psychiatric units, like those for patients leaving general hospitals, are disturbing and reflect concerning gaps in health-care quality. Pages and colleagues drilled down into data for 195 patients discharged from the psychiatric unit of a general hospital and compared those predictors and profiles to 2, 230 patients regularly discharged [2]. Patients received a comprehensive psychiatric assessment including scores on the Psychiatric Symptom Assessment Scale at admission and discharge. Surprisingly, there were no significant differences in discharge diagnoses. Patient demographics resembled those listed in Table 11.1 with more patients leaving AMA having a substance use diagnosis, using more psychoactive substances, being younger and male, being non-Caucasian, living alone, and having more prior hospitalizations. Male gender and younger age were, when analyzed, thought to be proxies for substance use. The authors also found that patients with less functional impairment and physical illness were more likely to leave AMA which may merely indicate it was easier physically for them to leave.

Follow-up of those patients who left AMA found that they stayed a shorter period in the hospital before discharge, had more severe psychiatric symptom scores at discharge, had higher rates of rehospitalization, and had higher utilization of inpatient psychiatric services even with consideration of the shorter stays.

Among the most tragic outcomes of AMA discharges from psychiatric units is suicide especially among patients with serious mental illnesses such as schizophrenia. Research into the relationship of diagnosis and prognosis in patients with schizophrenia, schizoaffective disorder, affective disorder, and borderline personality disorder who are discharged AMA found that patients with schizoaffective disorder were the most likely to commit suicide, while patients with unipolar mood disorder had the worst outcome [16].

Nearly 13,000 patients over nearly 20 years with an admission diagnosis of schizophrenia were examined in another study. Eight percent (674 patients) were discharged AMA, and their records were closely analyzed for rates of rehospitalization and mortality in comparison to patients with schizophrenia discharged with medical approval. The same predictive factors were identified: male, younger, and single. However, these patients had a shorter duration of illness suggesting hospitalization was not yet normalized for them, a hypothesis reinforced by the fact that 50% left within the first 2 weeks on the unit. Readmission rate and mortality as a result of both accidents and suicide were all higher than for those patients regularly discharged [17].

As Sclar and Robison point out, although the absolute number of patients with schizophrenia leaving AMA may seem insignificant in terms of negative impact on the health-care system, the cumulative effect represents a serious public health problem with considerable cost and loss of life, increased utilization of primary and specialty psychiatric care, and morbidity and mortality [18]. Their analysis of data from the 2004 US Healthcare Cost and Utilization Project Nationwide Inpatient Sample confirmed the risk factors already delineated but contrary to other studies did not find race to be a factor [2]. Length of stay in AMA versus approved discharges was 5 versus 8.7 days, respectively, and mean cost per day was $1886 in the AMA cohort compared to $1565 to those discharged when recommended.

Patient Rights and Psychiatrists' Duties

The data surveyed to this point on AMA discharges from psychiatric units generally reflect similar evidence about AMA discharges in medical populations covered in other chapters of this volume. And yet as Sclar comments, "Discharge against medical advice represents a challenge to the provision of care for patients with schizophrenia due to tension between patient's rights and psychiatrists' duties" [18]. This tension reflects the greater legal complexities of AMA discharges in psychiatry that distinguishes the ethical context of these clinical decisions when compared to that of other medical specialties. Consider a young male patient, Mr. S, with alcohol use disorder admitted to a general medical ward for alcohol withdrawal and a concern for acute pancreatitis. After the labs rule out pancreatitis and Mr. S is through the peak of withdrawal, he insists on leaving even though his physicians recommend he stay another day for further stabilization. The treatment team discharges Mr. S AMA.

Now add to this clinical picture that when initially evaluated in the emergency department that Mr. S instead of complaining of abdominal pain reports he is suicidal and so is admitted voluntarily to psychiatry. Several days after admission to the psychiatric unit, the acute withdrawal has resolved, but Mr. S continues to endorse suicidal ideation with a vague plan to "drink himself to death" and repeatedly demands to leave. The considerations facing the psychiatrist team at this juncture are more nuanced and complex than those facing general medical and surgical teams, and the exploration of these considerations will constitute the remainder of the chapter.

Parens Patriae and Police Powers

There is a fundamental conflict in US mental health policy, law, and ethics between a philosophy and practice founded on *parens patriae* and one grounded in police powers. Social, political, cultural, and economic forces are constantly adjusting the tension between the two approaches. *Parens patriae* which means literally in Latin "Father of the country" is beneficence based and is the position most clinicians favor. The philosophy and primary ethical justification for involuntary commitment under *parens patriae* is to provide needed psychiatric treatment to persons suffering from serious mental illness to restore their health and life. Under the philosophy of police powers endorsed by many legal professionals and civil rights advocates, the purpose of involuntary commitment is to prevent a patient from committing suicide or homicide or being utterly unable to care for themselves (i.e., "grave or passive neglect"). This is a rights and autonomy-based stance which holds that only the risk to self or others (John Stuart Mill's harm principle) ethically justifies the abrogation of individual privacy and liberty [19]. Patients who do not clearly and convincingly fit into these two boxes but have questionable decisional capacity and ability to function in the community and care for themselves and their families often fall into the cracks between these two positions. With each tragedy of the violent mentally ill strengthening the side of those arguing for stronger commitment laws, and every exploitation of the institutionalized mentally ill bolstering the side of voluntary admissions, public opinion and political agendas can shift.

One result of this constantly shifting policy pendulum that make AMA discharges in psychiatry so complicated is the spectrum of admission types from voluntary to commitment found in various states. In a 2014 article in the *Harvard Review of Psychiatry,* a group of experts in forensic psychiatry analyzed state statutes to ascertain patient's legal rights to request discharge when they have been voluntarily admitted to a psychiatric facility [20]. For all 50 states and the District of Columbia, the authors investigated three primary provisions: first, whether the law included a process to be followed when a voluntary patient

Table 11.2 Types of voluntary admissions

Type of admission	Restrictions on discharge
Pure informal voluntary	Discharged upon verbal request of patient; involuntary status cannot be legally pursued
Quasi-pure informal voluntary	May be required to give several days notification prior to being allowed to leave
	Can be placed on a psychiatric hold
	Petition for involuntary commitment can be filed
Formal or conditional voluntary admission	Patient must request discharge in writing
	Patient may be held for an evaluation period to determine if they can be discharged or be changed to involuntary status

requests discharge: second, the longest period a patient could be held against his will once a request to be discharged was lodged; and third, whether the statute included procedures to be followed if the treatment team decided to involuntarily commit a voluntary patient who requested discharge.

Types of Psychiatric Admissions

To fully appreciate the gravity of these limitations, it is important to understand that there are several types of voluntary admission to psychiatric hospitals each with its own legal implications for discharge. Table 11.2 summarizes the common designations [21].

Their analysis of state laws on voluntary discharge AMA shows that obstacles to the exercise of this right are common, technically complicated, and ethically significant. Forty-nine of the 51 statutes examined included provisions restricting the rights of voluntary patients to request discharge. For example, in 31 states the request for discharge must be made in writing. But the most formidable barrier to AMA discharge is the time limit state statutes impose. Forty-three state laws stipulate a maximal time a patient may be held against his will for observation. Seventy-two hours is the most frequent duration of this observation period, but as the authors underscore how these 72 h are defined varies leaving room for the voluntary patient to be held longer. Three states permit a facility to keep a patient for 5 days before discharging or committing while in only three states does the law actually allow a voluntary patient to be discharged immediately upon their request [20]. To this period of constrained confinement must be added the number of days the statute permits the treatment team to wait before they file the requisite petition for involuntary commitment extending from 24 h to 15 days with an average of 72 h [20].

The purpose of this observation period is for the treatment team to determine the patient's stability for release. At one end of the spectrum, the treatment team may find that Mr. S is at a high risk of suicide and hence cannot be discharged. Such a determination obligates the treatment team to place the patient on an official psychiatric hold and initiate the legal proceedings for involuntary commitment. At the other end of the spectrum of options, the psychiatric evaluation may find that Mr. S who is now no longer intoxicated or withdrawing is no acutely longer suicidal and can be safely discharged with the approval of the medical team to outpatient or residential care. It is between these two extremes that the law in many jurisdictions potentially compromises individual freedoms. The struggle to respect both the psychiatrists' duty of beneficence and the patient's right to autonomy are operative in this middle ground. Mr. S's assessment may indicate that although he no longer meets criteria for commitment, it would be more clinically appropriate for him to remain on the unit several more days to stabilize his depression. If Mr. S refuses this recommendation, then he would likely be discharged AMA. In view of the statutory delay and denial of an inpatient's initial request for discharge, the author's questioning of the authenticity of AMA discharge in psychiatry is legitimate [20].

Decisional Capacity, Informed Consent, and Coercion

This observation period and its attendant restrictions are not the only grounds upon which entire practice of voluntary admission (and by extension the AMA discharge) can be ethically criticized. The AMA discharge as conceptualized in general medicine is predicated on the patient's ability to provide informed consent. Indeed, clinicians and administrators alike often erroneously label AWOL or elopements as AMA discharges even though a cardinal element of the *AMA discharge* is an informed consent discussion with the responsible practitioner. If there is no "medical advice" from the clinician, then there can be no "discharge against it."

Garakani et al. also scrutinize the validity of the AMA discharge in psychiatry in terms of a lack of authentic informed consent [18]. Given the ambiguity and granularity of the regulations governing voluntary admissions, it is reasonable to believe that Mr. S will not grasp the conditional nature of the voluntary admission to which he consents in the emergency department. When the mental health professional, often a mid-level provider or a resident physician, in large academic medical centers or community hospitals offers Mr. S the choice, he may well not have had full decision-making capacity secondary to alcohol intoxication, alcohol withdrawal, or both. It is equally likely that the mental health professional herself even accurately comprehends and can explain in language Mr. S relates to the restrictions imposed on a patient-initiated discharge from a voluntary admission to psychiatry. For example, a study with North Carolina psychiatric residents identified lack of knowledge of the commitment parameters in their state [22], and another study identified that patients are more likely to leave AMA when residents are involved in their care [23]. These two findings underscore the need to educate house officers and attendings in the laws of their practice locality. Thus, the three primary elements required legally and ethically for informed consent to admission (sufficient information, decisional capacity, and voluntarism) are all at best inadequate and at worse barely existent [24].

This questioning of the capacity to provide informed consent for admission and by logical corollary discharge has gone all the way to the US Supreme Court in the

1990 case of *Zinermon v. Burch* [25]. Darrel Burch was found lost, confused, and injured on a Florida highway. Transported to an emergency department, he was diagnosed with schizophrenia and then transferred to the Florida State Hospital. Mr. Burch signed forms requesting admission to the hospital and consenting to treatment at the facility. Yet staff at the time of his intake evaluation described the patient as obviously delusional, "upon his arrival at ACMHS, Burch was hallucinating, confused, psychotic, and believed he was "in heaven" [25].

Although diagnosed as acutely psychotic, Mr. Burch was held voluntarily at the state hospital for 5 months without a court hearing. Once discharged he took legal action against the hospital, its leadership, and his physicians, claiming that due to florid psychosis he was without capacity to consent to voluntary admission and so was deprived of the due process protections he should have received as an incapable patient admitted involuntarily.

The case eventually went to the Supreme Court which decided in the patient's favor, ruling that the state had an obligation to evaluate the capacity to consent of voluntary patients to ensure they were not hospitalized against their will without a judicial hearing. The Court's opinion emphasizes the inherent connection between the ability to consent for admission and to request discharge:

> Indeed, the very nature of mental illness makes it foreseeable that a person needing mental health care will be unable to understand any proffered 'explanation and disclosure of the subject matter' of the forms that person is asked to sign, and will be unable to make a 'knowing and willful decision' whether to consent to admission. A person who is willing to sign forms but is incapable of making an informed decision is, by the same token, unlikely to benefit from the voluntary patient's statutory right to request discharge. [25]

The scope of the ruling was limited in that it applied only to states that already required informed consent for voluntary psychiatric admission. These jurisdictions the high court held must develop reasonable procedures for screening the capacity of patients consenting to voluntary admission. In response to the ruling, the American Psychiatric Association issued guidelines for ensuring that patients have the capacity to consent to voluntary admission. Given that the majority of states do not legally require consent for voluntary psychiatric admission, that the court ruling did not actually stipulate a specific protocol for these screening evaluations, and that the APA made recommendations not mandates, the court decision did little to strengthen the legal safeguards for a patient with questionable capacity who nonetheless agrees to voluntary admission [26]. This legal gap in obtaining informed consent for admission yet permitting restrictions on a patient's right to voluntary discharge is among the most ethically problematic aspects of AMA discharges from inpatient psychiatry.

In clinical practice and even in some mental health hearings, this not infrequently means that a patient with psychosis or dementia who knows "he is going to the hospital for help" may be considered a voluntary admission. When this inadequacy is combined with the implicit, and at times explicit, coercion with which the choice between involuntary and voluntary admission is often presented to patients [27], it becomes difficult to not question the extent to which a patient can be ethically discharged *AMA* from a psychiatric facility. Certainly, mental health professionals can and will continue to make this clinical determination and utilize the term AMA discharge to describe the conditions of discharge from inpatient psychiatric treatment, but the voluntariness of the admission and its ethical impact on requests for AMA discharge remain areas of uncertainty deserving of more consideration.

Consider the following case:

Ms. R is a patient with bipolar I disorder with psychotic features who the police apprehended while she was riding her bicycle naked down a major highway singing she is winning the Tour De France. The police transports her to the psychiatric emergency department of an academic medical center on a busy holiday weekend where a hurried and harried resident who recognizes her from prior admissions says, "Ms. R., you can either come in involuntarily or voluntarily, what is it going to be this time? I am giving you the choice but if you don't come in on your own I will have to take you to court for a commitment and that means you will likely stay longer." Ms. R asks, "If I go voluntarily, how long do I have to stay?Because I need to find someone to take care of my dog; I left her in the yard before I went to the race." The resident, who knows a voluntary admission is much less work for his team, says, "If you are voluntary, you can leave whenever you want." Ms. R reasonably, but reluctantly, agrees to voluntary admission. There is no mention of the conditions and limitations under which Ms. R will be granted a discharge, ostensibly to care for her dog. Is it not only the style and tone in which these options are framed that make the patient's choice between voluntary and involuntary a "false" one? While some mental health ethicists would claim this is an inherently coercive situation, others would contend that presenting the option of involuntary admission as one alternative is if done respectfully and compassionately is an essential aspect of the informed consent process for admission [28]. If the resident was to reframe and say "I have a duty to keep you safe and help you feel better. I don't think this can happen outside the hospital as ill as you are right now. I respect that you may not want to come into the ward but you have the right to make your own decision. If you choose not to be admitted, then I may need to make the decision to involuntarily admit as the best way to keep you safe and get well so you can take care of your dog."

Empirical studies suggest that from the patient's perspective, it is not the voluntary/involuntary status that is the measure of coercion so much as the patient's sense the admission is fair and they have access to due process [29]. Although the research has not yet been done, the same considerations may well be applicable to the management of AMA discharges particularly in those jurisdictions that permit a waiting period for evaluation. When discussing coercion, it must be recognized that legal coercion may be the most direct and transparent of the pressures pushing a patient toward voluntary hospitalization. Other constraints such as family ultimatums, threats from employers, criminal justice consequences, or clinician "persuasion" may be more insidious and indirect. Conversely, many of these same considerations constrain the ability of patients to complete treatment episodes and hence influence requests for AMA discharge even when the patient knows that in leaving they are acting against their own best therapeutic interest [14]. The body of literature pertaining to patient perceptions of coercion in psychiatric admission may thus be a potential resource for understanding patient-initiated requests for discharge and how to most positively manage them.

Encounters such as this which likely occur hundreds of times a day in US emergency rooms and inpatient units in mental health facilities across the country are the reason Garakani and colleagues recommend ethical standards for informed consent to voluntary admission be instituted that could then inform and reform changes in state laws. Their proposal would address the infringements of autonomy and breach of trust, however, well-intentioned, evinced in the case of Ms. R. In addition, standards would equip voluntary patients with the same legal protections and procedural fairness that a hearing before a mental health court or other judiciary body ensures to patients admitted involuntarily. In contrast to the first scenario played out between the resident and Ms. R, commitment proceedings involve due process with legal representation granted to the patient, often the involvement of a patient advocate and a judicial review of the psychiatrist's clinical justification of the deprivation of liberty [28].

Reform of voluntary admission in accordance with the legal and ethical principles of informed consent is therefore the sine qua non of a meaningful AMA discharge in psychiatry. The ability of a patient with decision-making capacity diagnosed with a mental health disorder to be treated as the equal of a capable patient with a medical condition is critical. Psychiatric patients who refuse to remain in the hospital can only be assured that the patient is granted an unrestricted and informed right to request and be granted discharge as is already established in medical hospitalizations.

Voluntary psychiatric admissions are among the most therapeutic interventions in psychiatry. Voluntary admissions are a triumph of the movement toward destigmatization and civil rights in mental health care. While maximizing the healing potential of the therapeutic alliance, voluntary admission minimizes the intrusive nature of recourse to the courts and the dehumanization of care that are all too frequent consequences of involuntary commitment. But just as yes is meaningless without the possibility of no, so discharge AMA does not exist for psychiatric patients without their being told the truth about the admission and the circumstances under which they may or may not be permitted to leave if they desire to do so.

Liability

The foremost concern in the minds of many experienced and thoughtful psychiatrists and other mental health professionals reading this argument is that of liability. What happens if when Mr. S is in one of the few states without an observation period, clearly does not meet requirement for inpatient admission, leaves AMA, and goes out and commits suicide? What if Ms. R when she learns she cannot immediately go home to her dog refuses voluntary admission and yet not being an imminent danger to herself or others does not meet the state criteria for involuntary admission and so deteriorates further? Many clinicians, because of concerns over liability, work to ensure both patients sign AMA forms. Given the current debate on the value of a signed AMA form in conferring protection for a provider from legal liability and the suggestion that it has an adverse impact on the treatment relationship, still there is almost no research on the utility and efficacy of a signed AMA form in psychiatry. Thought leaders also differ in their estimation of the protective purpose of the signed form. Appelbaum and Gutheil modestly endorse the usefulness of the AMA form:

> These patient-initiated discharges often referred to as *against medical advice* or *AMA*. Strictly speaking however, this is not always the case, as there are instances in which, for a variety of clinical reasons, the patient's caregivers acquiesce in the decision to leave. When the discharge occurs over the strenuous opposition of the clinical staff, it is sometimes useful to acknowledge this by having the noncommittable patient sign a second form, similar to that used in medical hospitals, indicating that the patient is aware of the grounds for the hospital's opposition to her departure. In addition, to the positive clinical effects of such a procedure, the additional documentation may be useful in the event that harm befalls the patient or a third party as a result of the premature cessation of inpatient treatment. [21]

Gerbasi and Simon are more cautionary:

> It is unlikely that the plaintiff's not having a signed form will be proof of negligence, but, a signed AMA form will not be especially protective either; the psychiatrist's mere possession of a patient's signed AMA form is not a talisman that magically wards off the threat of litigation. The form merely documents a patient's awareness, although not necessarily his or her meaningful understanding, of the psychiatrists' warning about the risks of premature discharge. It should be the clinical staff—and not the AMA form—that provides the patient with information concerning the potential consequences and risks of being discharged AMA. [30]

The general consensus among risk managers and hospital attorneys is that what is protective is not a signed form but the conduct and documentation in the medical record of the informed consent discussion it codifies. Two reviews of malpractice litigation related to AMA discharges from psychiatry units [30, 31] offer guidance for the mental health professional faced with this difficult dilemma. Devitt and Dewan outline two cases that occurred in Veterans Administration (VA) hospitals. In one instance, the patient committed suicide within hours of AMA discharge after only 1 day in the hospital [32]. The second case, the day the patient was discharged AMA he stabbed a police officer [33]. In both cases, the court found that the defendant physicians were not negligent. The authors draw several hortatory lessons from their analysis [31, 34]. First and foremost, a psychiatrist is far more likely to be successfully sued for the patient who leaves AMA and harms or kills himself or someone else than for seeking involuntary commitment. The salient caveat is that if a psychiatrist cogently and conscientiously documents the reasons a patient does not meet her state's criteria for involuntary admission, they have a far greater chance of prevailing in court if a suicide, homicide, or serious decompensation later occurs [30]. We have already seen that there is potential legal jeopardy in holding a "voluntary" patient requesting to leave without recourse to commitment proceedings. Devitt and Dewan's comment that "Good clinical practice and thorough documentation remain the best legal protection. Discharging a patient against medical advice may provide partial protection, but it is not a royal road to legal immunity" would be an apt motto for every psychiatric hospitalist to post on the wall of their office [31]. And when the psychiatrist has serious and persistent concerns that discharging the patient AMA is dangerous even if the case for involuntary commitment criteria is not particularly strong, the safest and most just course is often to move to commit the patient and allow the court to decide.

Tarasoff and AMA Discharge

In the back of the mind of almost every American psychiatrist, considering an AMA discharge is the specter of the *Tarasoff* case and the duty to protect it established in the professional standard of care in psychiatry [35] as shown in the following case.

Sgt. J is a career police officer who claims he is being forced out of the department unfairly several years before retirement. After his wife found him with his service revolver in his mouth one night and at her insistence, he requests voluntary admission for treatment of major depressive disorder with homicidal and suicidal ideation. After a week of antidepressant medication and psychotherapy as well as the support of the inpatient milieu, Sgt. J is no longer experiencing persistent thoughts of harming himself. Yet he does continue to have some intrusive impulses to shoot the police lieutenant he believes is responsible for his suspension from the force. He has no plan or timeline to shoot the officer and for now states he will see how the appeal goes. Sgt. J requests to be discharged so he can meet with his police union representative and attorneys to prepare for the appeal which he feels he cannot adequately do while inpatient. The psychiatrist believes Sgt. J is just starting to respond to treatment and needs another week of hospitalization before discharge to outpatient follow-up. Although the psychiatrist recognizes that Sgt. J does not meet his state's criteria for commitment of imminent harm, he does believe that in the language of Tarasoff the police lieutenant is an identifiable victim and Sgt. J acting violently toward him is foreseeable. Thus, the psychiatrist believes he could be held accountable if Sgt. J harms the lieutenant. The Tarasoff ruling is often misunderstood to require a duty to warn when it really imposed a duty to protect [36]. Hospitalizing Mr. J satisfied that duty to protect the object of harm. But with the patient's impending discharge, the psychiatrist determined that honoring that duty to protect will now require warning the police lieutenant of the potential threat to his life. Tarasoff in general provides immunity to the mental health professional carrying out this duty to warn in good faith, but therapeutically it is prudent to disclose this necessity to Sgt. J and to try and involve him in the warning. Sgt. J may well experience this duty to protect others as therapeutic and change his mind about the discharge or more probably perceive it as coercive and angrily leave the unit ironically increasing his likelihood of violence.

Managed Care

Making the clinical decision whether to discharge or commit is never easy even for a seasoned psychiatrist. However, an even more distressing conundrum is when both patient and clinician believe that the patient is not sufficiently stable for discharge, but the insurance company or other third party makes an administrative decision that the patient no longer needs inpatient treatment. This rise of managed care in the 1980s and the emphasis on utilization review in the recent years as forms of cost-control and efficiency improvement have confronted mental health professionals especially in the private and community sectors with new ethical challenges. Psychiatrists caught between the demands of third parties and the clinical needs of patients must always ally with, and defend, the good of the patient even though such fiduciary action may place their own livelihood at risk. This risk can be minimized if psychiatrist, and patient or family if appropriate, file timely and clinically solid appeals to the insurance company or utilization reviewer. Studies have found that desperate practitioners may with the best of intentions attempt to deceive third parties to gain approval of additional hospital days [37]. While this is understandable, the more legally and ethically sound strategy is for the treating professional to continue to provide reasoned and accurate documentation of the patient's clinical condition and indices for *inpatient* treatment along with rationales for why this care cannot be successfully and safely delivered outside the hospital setting [38].

Preventive Ethics and Best Practices

Much of this chapter has perforce been occupied with surveying the epidemiology of AMA discharges in inpatient psychiatry, distinguishing the legal, political, social, and ethical aspects that separate AMA discharges in inpatient psychiatry from those in other areas of health care. In this final section of the chapter, we draw on this material to inform proposals for preventive ethics methods and best clinical practices for improving the management of AMA discharges in inpatient psychiatry. These strategies are designed to predict requests to leave when possible, reduce discharges AMA when feasible, and minimize the adverse health and health services outcomes of such discharges at every reasonable opportunity.

Research on AMA discharges in medicine and psychiatry sketch a picture of the demographics and circumstances of patients leaving AMA from inpatient psychiatry units [15], and yet there are relatively few studies that have utilized this information to design performance improvement projects although the data offer discernable targets. One of the only articles reporting on an intervention found that offering a patient advocate to champion the autonomy and rights of patients, substantially, reduced AMA discharges from a private psychiatric hospital [39]. Several of these articles cited here offer endorsable recommendations, with the limitation that very few have empirical support.

Staff in both the emergency department and the inpatient unit should be edu-cated about the types of clinical scenarios when patients may be more likely to initi-ate AMA discharges while avoiding profiling. Louks [40] stresses the near prophetic value of prior AMA discharges, and this would seem a prime target for intensive case management. Similarly, the temporal conditions under which patients are more likely to request discharge have been identified and extra attention paid to weekends, nights, and holidays when there may be not only be less staff but more staff who are unfamiliar with the patient. Detailed documentation from the regular inpatient teams including discharge plans can help an on-call team both anticipate and handle constructively AMA discharge requests.

One promising intervention would be the design of an orientation protocol. Research has shown that the seeds of AMA discharges are often planted in the admission process. Part of the shared decision-making discussion regarding vol-untary admission even if it eventuates in an involuntary decision should be a description of the psychiatric ward and its routine. This is especially critical for patients who have never been psychiatrically hospitalized before. Such an orienta-tion can set the expectation that patients will be treated with dignity and invited to participate in treatment planning to the full extent their condition and treatment allows. Beck and colleagues underscore the first week of admission as a crucial time in which especially emotionally dysregulated patients may ask to leave. Increased attention to the building and maintaining the therapeutic alliance during these periods of heighted vulnerability may be efficacious [12]. Substance use disorders are ubiquitous in studies of AMA predictive factors, and the endemic failure to properly diagnose and treat them in a timely manner is a system-wide problem that, if addressed, has real potential to decrease patient-initiated dis-charges [41].

The need to empower these patients caught in the "revolving door" of our frag-mented underfunded health-care system has been neglected [42]. Depending on the nature of the relationship to the patient, families may be enlisted to encourage the patient to remain in the hospital. Patient permission should in general be sought to communicate with family members, but there may be exigencies in which the safety of the patient may outweigh or validate the violation of confidentiality.

Patients can be encouraged to complete psychiatric advance directives (PADs) that appoint proxy decision-makers in those jurisdictions where this is permitted and provide instructions to proxies and physicians regarding their wishes should they request AMA discharge. Unfortunately, in many states patient preferences expressed in PADs even regarding psychiatric admission have been legally over-ridden even when in the clinical judgment of the treatment team continued inpa-tient care is psychiatrically indicated [43]. It also true that Ms. R could have completed a PAD when psychiatrically stable and, yet when manic or depressed, she could rescind her own preferences and contravene her own values requiring legal recourse to keep her in the hospital, a catch-22 called the Ulysses contract in the ethics literature. But even despite the legal loopholes, the need for additional court hearings to try and break the Ulysses contract, PADs remain worthwhile tools to promote shared decision-making with untapped potential to avoid AMA discharge [44].

The therapeutic alliance that is at the heart of mental health care may well be the single most powerful means of decreasing the number of AMA discharges and ameliorating their outcomes. Psychotherapeutically, AMA discharges represent either thwarted therapeutic relationships or abrupt ruptures in an alliance that are not repaired or sadly in some instances, not repairable. Negative perceptions such as when patients view the milieu as punitive and staff perceive the patient to be angry are far more likely to result in leaving AMA likely because of an atmosphere of mutual distrust and dislike. Among the most interesting psychodynamic formulation is the suggestion that AMA discharges may have different meanings for the patient depending on the diagnosis that has clinical relevance for outcome and follow-up. McGlashan and Heinssen suggest that in borderline patients, AMA discharges can represent a healthy assertion of autonomy when the patient feels the episode of emotional dysregulation that brought them to the hospital has resolved. Where the AMA departure of a patient with schizoaffective disorder or major depression may suggest increased hopelessness and a higher risk of suicide, warranting close follow-up and suicide prevention plans [16]. Understanding the meaning of the request for the patient can mediate even a fractured relationship between provider and patient. Remembering that even forensic masters cannot reliably predict violence particularly in the longer term brings into relief the practical obstacles in informing patients of the risks of AMA discharge and thus truthfully conveying the benefits of remaining the hospital. Returning to the patient's personal goals for the initial hospitalization such as relief of terrifying paranoia, ability to obtain an apartment, and finding a more tolerable medication can establish a common ground for negotiation. Building on these goals, reasonable efforts to minimize negative staff interactions, offering/changing medications to relieve symptoms, granting requested privileges, or recruiting an outpatient psychiatrist the patient trusts or a friend they rely upon in the community, may circumvent even if temporarily the demand for discharge facilitating additional space to evaluate and time to plan a safer and more appropriate discharge. In the end, for some astute patients whose insight is that hospitalization is exacerbating the course of illness, a humanistic discharge to outpatient care and home that may be beneficial and better promote the patient's mental health.

Brooks' review cited earlier is one of the few articles to concentrate on *provider factors* in AMA discharge that are low-hanging fruit ripe for positive change [10]. Staff can be trained to watch and listen for the sights and sounds of patient dissatisfaction with treatment, protestations of not getting better, and feelings of not being respected or ignored that smolder until they ignite in a request for discharge. Empathic validation, consistent fair limit setting, and personalized proactive care implemented through enhanced facilitation techniques and communication skills are both teachable and effective. Inpatient unit medical directors and nurse managers can model and mentor these superior interpersonal skills for staff setting a tone that line staff will imitate. These leaders also need support. Access to senior clinical colleagues as well as available ethics and legal consultants who offer not only solidarity in the solitude of these weighty decisions but also the ability to generate previously unappreciated alternatives can correct for the myopia of burn-out that can lead to professional errors in judgment.

Finally, just as with discharges AMA from the medical wards of general hospitals, practitioners must even on a holiday weekend or the middle of the night do their best to arrange suitable follow-up, discharge medications, facilitation of a return to the hospital, or accessing other mental health care if the patient so desires and referral to a safe disposition. Even if a court did not find these steps reflective of the good faith intentions and judgment of the psychiatrist, not taking them is neither good clinical practice nor ethically justifiable.

Conclusion

The review of epidemiological literature on AMA discharges from psychiatric hospitals presented in this chapter exhibits similar patient features and environmental patterns as AMA discharges from general medical hospitals. However, the thesis of this chapter is that the hallmark of AMA psychiatric discharges is a complex and ambiguous combination of ethical issues and legal considerations that distinguish AMA discharges in psychiatry. Having reviewed the political and philosophical background of psychiatric hospitalization, current debates regarding decisional capacity, informed consent, and coercion in voluntary admission were analyzed. The legal liability concerns of psychiatrists confronted with patient-initiated requests for discharge and their clinical implications were critically examined. Based on the literature and analysis, the chapter proffered recommendations for preventive ethics strategies and best practices to reduce the frequency and improve the quality of AMA discharges from psychiatry. The discussion of AMA discharges from inpatient psychiatric facilities presented here highlights many unexplored clinical and ethical issues that would benefit from future empirical research.

References

1. Molnar G, Keitner L, Swindall L. Medicolegal problems of elopement from psychiatric units. J Forensic Sci. 1985;30(1):44–9.
2. Pages KP, Russo JE, Wingerson DK, Ries RK, Roy-Byrne PP, Cowley DS. Predictors and outcome of discharge against medical advice from the psychiatric units of a general hospital. Psychiatr Serv. 1998;49(9):1187–92.
3. Blader JC. Acute inpatient care for psychiatric disorders in the United States, 1996 through 2007. Arch Gen Psychiatry. 2011;68(12):1276–83.
4. Haupt DN, Ehrlich SM. The impact of a new state commitment law on psychiatric patient careers. Hosp Community Psychiatry. 1980;31(11):745–51.
5. Babalola O, Gormez V, Alwan NA, Johnstone P, Sampson S. Length of hospitalisation for people with severe mental illness. Cochrane Database Syst Rev. 2014;1:CD000384.

6. Chandrasena R. Premature discharges: a comparative study. Can J Psychiatr. 1987;32(4): 259–63.
7. Alfandre DJ. "I'm going home": discharges against medical advice. Mayo Clin Proc. 2009;84(3):255–60.
8. LaWall JS, Jones R. Discharges from a ward against medical advice: search for a profile. Hosp Community Psychiatry. 1980;31(6):415–6.
9. Senior N, Kibbee P. Can we predict the patient who leaves against medical advice: the search for a method. Psychiatr Hosp. 1986;17(1):33–6.
10. Brook M, Hilty DM, Liu W, Hu R, Frye MA. Discharge against medical advice from inpatient psychiatric treatment: a literature review. Psychiatr Serv. 2006;57(8):1192–8.
11. Yong TY, Fok JS, Hakendorf P, Ben-Tovim D, Thompson CH, Li JY. Characteristics and outcomes of discharges against medical advice among hospitalised patients. Intern Med J. 2013;43(7):798–802.
12. Beck NC, Shekim W, Gilbert F, Fraps C. A cross-validation of factors predictive of AMA discharge. Hosp Community Psychiatry. 1983;34(1):69–70.
13. Hayat AA, Ahmed MM, Minhas FA. Patients leaving against medical advice: an inpatient psychiatric hospital-based study. J Coll Physicians Surg Pak. 2013;23(5):342–6.
14. Akhtar S, Helfrich J, Mestayer RF. AMA discharge from a psychiatric inpatient unit. Int J Soc Psychiatry. 1981;27(2):143–50.
15. Dalrymple AJ, Fata M. Cross-validating factors associated with discharges against medical advice. Can J Psychiatr. 1993;38(4):285–9.
16. McGlashan TH, Heinssen RK. Hospital discharge status and long-term outcome for patients with schizophrenia, schizoaffective disorder, borderline personality disorder, and unipolar affective disorder. Arch Gen Psychiatry. 1988;45(4):363–8.
17. Valevski A, Zalsman G, Tsafrir S, Lipschitz-Elhawi R, Weizman A, Shohat T. Rate of readmission and mortality risks of schizophrenia patients who were discharged against medical advice. Eur Psychiatry. 2012;27(7):496–9.
18. Sclar DA, Robison LM. Hospital admission for schizophrenia and discharge against medical advice in the United States. Prim Care Companion J Clin Psychiatry. 2010;12(2): e1–e6.
19. Appelbaum PS, Gutheil TG. Legal issues in emergency psychiatry. In: Appelbaum PS, Gutheil TG, editors. Clinical handbook of psychiatry & the law. Philadelphia: Lippincott, Williams & WIlkins; 2007.
20. Garakani A, Shalenberg E, Burstin SC, Weintraub Brendel R, Appel JM. Voluntary psychiatric hospitalization and patient-driven requests for discharge: a statutory review and analysis of implications for the capacity to consent to voluntary hospitalization. Harv Rev Psychiatry. 2014;22(4):241–9.
21. Appelbaum PS, Gutheil TG. Legal issues in inpatient psychiatry. In: Appelbaum PS, Gutheil TG, editors. Clinical handbook of psychiatry & the law. Philadelphia: Lippincott, Williams & Wilkins; 2007.
22. Kaufman AR, Way B. North Carolina resident psychiatrists knowledge of the commitment statutes: do they stray from the legal standard in the hypothetical application of involuntary commitment criteria? Psychiatry Q. 2010;81(4):363–7.
23. Greenwald AF, Bartemeier LH. Psychiatric discharges against medical advice. Arch Gen Psychiatry. 1963;8:117–9.
24. Appelbaum PS. Clinical practice. Assessment of patients' competence to consent to treatment. N Engl J Med. 2007;357(18):1834–40.
25. Zinermon v. Burch. 1990, U.S. p. 113.
26. Appelbaum PS. Voluntary hospitalization and due process: the dilemma of Zinermon v. Burch Hosp Comm Psychiatr. 1990;41(10):1059–60.
27. O'Donoghue B, Roche E, Shannon S, Lyne J, Madigan K, Feeney L. Perceived coercion in voluntary hospital admission. Psychiatry Res. 2014;215(1):120–6.
28. Stone DH. The benefits of voluntary inpatient psychiatric hospitalization: myth or reality? Boston Univ Public Interest Law J. 1999;9(1):25–52.

29. Lidz CW, Hoge SK, Gardner W, Bennett NS, Monahan J, Mulvey EP, et al. Perceived coercion in mental hospital admission. Pressures and process. Arch Gen Psychiatr. 1995;52(12): 1034–9.
30. Gerbasi JB, Simon RI. Patients' rights and psychiatrists' duties: discharging patients against medical advice. Harv Rev Psychiatry. 2003;11(6):333–43.
31. Devitt PJ, Devitt AC, Dewan M. An examination of whether discharging patients against medical advice protects physicians from malpractice charges. Psychiatr Serv. 2000;51(7): 899–902.
32. Solbrig v. the United States of America, in Lexis 2201. 1995, U.S. Dist.
33. Kelly v. the United States of America and John Doe, John Roe, & John Shoe, in Lexis 2201. 1987, Civil Action 86–2864.
34. Devitt PJ, Devitt AC, Dewan M. Does identifying a discharge as "against medical advice" confer legal protection? J Fam Pract. 2000;49(3):224–7.
35. Tarasoff v. Regents of University of California 1976, Cal.3d. p. 425.
36. Knoll JL. The psychiatrist's duty to protect. CNS Spectr. 2015;20(3):215–22.
37. Dwyer J, Shih A. The ethics of tailoring the patient's chart [see comments]. Psychiatr Serv. 1998;49(10):1309–12.
38. Simon RI. Psychiatrists' duties in discharging sicker and potentially violent inpatients in the managed care era. Psychiatr Serv. 1998;49(1):62–7.
39. Targum SD, Capodanno AE, Hoffman HA, Foudraine C. An intervention to reduce the rate of hospital discharges against medical advice. Am J Psychiatry. 1982;139(5):657–9.
40. Louks J, Mason J, Backus F. AMA discharges: prediction and treatment outcome. Hosp Community Psychiatry. 1989;40(3):299–301.
41. Ti L, Ti L. Leaving the hospital against medical advice among people who use illicit drugs: a systematic review. Am J Public Health. 2015;105(12):e53–9.
42. Chandrasena R, Miller WC. Discharges AMA and AWOL: a new "revolving door syndrome". Psychiatr J Univ Ott. 1988;13(3):154–7.
43. Swanson JW, McCrary SV, Swartz MS, Elbogen EB, Van Dorn RA. Superseding psychiatric advance directives: ethical and legal considerations. J Am Acad Psychiatry Law. 2006;34(3):385–94.
44. Brock DW. A proposal for the use of advance directives in the treatment of incompetent mentally ill persons. Bioethics. 1993;7(2–3):247–56.

Index